AF556728

Health Outcomes and the Pakistani Population

Health Outcomes and the Pakistani Population

By

Ikhlaq Din

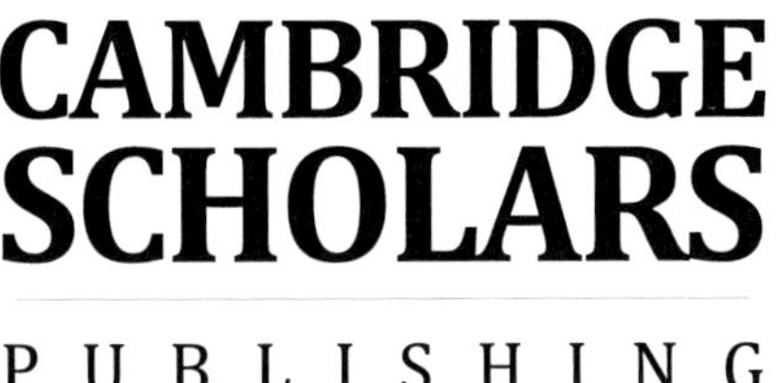

Health Outcomes and the Pakistani Population,
by Ikhlaq Din

This book first published 2014

Cambridge Scholars Publishing

12 Back Chapman Street, Newcastle upon Tyne, NE6 2XX, UK

British Library Cataloguing in Publication Data
A catalogue record for this book is available from the British Library

ISBN (10): 1-4438-6134-0, ISBN (13): 978-1-4438-6134-2

TABLE OF CONTENTS

CHAPTER ONE

INTRODUCTION

Background

This book examines dietary habits and physical activity among older Pakistani people in Mirpur, Pakistan. It explores how diet has changed over time in Pakistan. It also explores the ways in which older Pakistani people participate in physical activities. This was carried out by conducting in-depth semi-structured interviews with residents in Mirpur, Pakistan.

The research reveals some unique insights into the Pakistani community. By exploring physical activities among Pakistanis, the author was able to explore perceptions held by the 'community'; these include cultural norms and values that dictate whether individuals are allowed to participate or not, for example 'restrictions' placed on females that prevent them from freely engaging in physical activity.

This research shows that, although some older female respondents said they would like to participate in physical activity, the overriding cultural norms dictate that only a very small minority of females were allowed to do so. Practices varied mainly along the lines of socioeconomic background and all the females who said they participated in physical activity were from middle-class backgrounds.

In addition, this book has several chapters on methods, which can act as a reference guide to researchers who wish to examine a minority ethnic community, in this case the Pakistanis.

The researcher

Research is usually conducted by way of personal interest for the author(s). My parents were born in the district of Mirpur and I grew up hearing stories of family 'get togethers' where food played a pivotal role in family life and functions. Food brought individuals and families together. Whilst I was growing up, I heard stories of how meals were cooked on a 'mega scale' for all the 'family' to enjoy ('family' included parents, siblings, grandparents, uncles, aunts, close relatives and friends), where they would sit together on the floor and enjoy a well-earned evening meal after a hard day's work.

The important link to bringing families and individuals together was food. Food brought everyone together, whether it was for the main evening meal, to celebrate a birth or marriage, or even to mourn a death. Food was served in a celebratory manner and they were thankful for what the family could afford, however much or little.

It was a time to relax and enjoy family life. I also heard stories about the daily struggles and hardships of everyday life for most Pakistanis during and after Independence in 1947, which later provided the impetus to immigrate to the UK when the opportunity arose (discussed later). What little food families had was shared.

During an earlier visit to Pakistan, I observed that most families I visited were consuming traditional foods, e.g. curries (meat and veg) and rotis, mostly due to limited finances. However, during my last visit I observed an increasing number of people were eating out in the bazaar and consuming a vast array of foods, particularly fried foods, sweet desserts and drinking an array of fizzy drinks. Much of this was linked to an increase in the family's financial status. There is a link between an increase in spending on food items and family status. For the purposes of this research, there was a clear division between those families who could afford to eat what they liked, as often as and when they wished, compared to many Pakistani families who were on very limited incomes struggling to make ends meet.

CHAPTER TWO

HEALTH OF PAKISTANIS

This chapter covers a preliminary literature search on dietary habits of Pakistanis and South Asians. Three of the world's ten most populated countries are located in South Asia. The problems seem to be different from those of the developed world, with rapidly changing socioeconomic circumstances, increasing urbanisation and longevity, changes in dietary patterns and a decrease in mortality from infectious diseases, which have made chronic illnesses of old age, such as cardiovascular disease and strokes, an important areas of focus. The risk factors for diabetes are well-established including obesity, smoking, hypertension and family history of diabetes (Fawwad et al., 2013).

The Commission on Health Research for Development (1990) stressed the importance of national health research in developing countries. It estimated that at around 2% of the national budget should be made available for health research, which it considered to be paramount for developing countries (Hyder et al., 2003). A literature search for purposes of this book showed an increasing number of studies being conducted in Pakistan around dietary habits and physical activity. This is important in order to understand health issues and to develop interventions that tackle unhealthy behaviours. There is a need to understand geographical differences because experience suggests that dietary behaviour varies enormously.

Asian diet

The dietary customs of people of South Asian origin living in Britain are important determinants of health (Simmons and Williams, 1997). They found that those of South Asian origin ate fewer meals per day than European participants, but ate more fruit. Further, South Asians had their evening meal 2-3 hours later than their European counterparts.

Research shows that the Asian diet can have an effect on conditions such as coronary heart disease (McKeigue et al., 1985), non-insulin dependent diabetes mellitus (McKeigue et al., 1991), rickets, anaemia

(Robertson, 1982) and eye conditions such as cataracts (Thompson, 1991). Sheikh and Thomas (1994) argue that the Asian population has a diet which differs from the indigenous white population; for example, Asian populations often have a vegetarian diet which has been linked to the development of rickets, iron deficiency B12, folic acid anaemia and, more recently, cataracts.

Råberg et al. (2010) found the most important barriers to healthy dietary changes were preferences of children and other family members and perceived expectations during social gatherings. They found the perceived pressure was strong when women were trying to change to more vegetables, lentils and fish and to use less oil in cooking.

Obesity epidemic

Obesity is considered a global epidemic (Ishaque et al., 2012). It has become a problem of public health magnitude. It is associated with substantial economic burden, not only in the developed countries but also in the developing countries (Afzal, 2004).

There is an enormous amount of literature that examines obesity in Pakistani populations, with an increasing number of studies being conducted in Pakistan. This is essential in order to understand the increasing problem of obesity and the impact this will have on the health budget in Pakistan.

Obesity is an emerging problem in Pakistan. Obesity in childhood and adolescence is of concern because it is an important predictor of adult obesity (Ishaque et al., 2012). The study by Warraich (2009), which examined the prevalence of childhood obesity, found that 52% were found to be overweight and 34% of all children were normal. Of the population, 6% were obese and 8% overweight. Interestingly, of all obese children, 70% were from the higher socioeconomic status and a higher number of them ate meat every day compared to children from lower socioeconomic groups (65% versus 33% respectively). This is similar to the findings by Ishaque et al. (2012), who found the frequency of overweight and obese children was high in children from higher socioeconomic status.

Imam et al. (2000) studied 869 people visiting Lahore General Hospital (Pakistan). They were evaluated for their body mass index (BMI) in a random fashion to determine the prevalence of obesity. They found that 170 subjects had a BMI of 25 to 30 in a pre-obesity range of BMI and 51 subjects were in an obese range of 30 to 40. They suggested that urgent public health measures be taken to prevent a rise in obesity in the suburbs of Lahore.

The study by Nanan (2002), which examined the health outcomes associated with overweight and obesity, suggests that, in South Asia, including Pakistan, social and environmental changes are occurring rapidly, with increasing urbanisation, changing lifestyles, high energy density of diets and reduced physical activity, all contributing to an increase in obesity. Nanan found that the prevalence of obesity in the 25-44 age group in rural areas of Pakistan was 9% for men and 14% for women. By contrast, in the urban areas, the prevalence was 22% for men and 37% for women. For the 45-64 age group, the prevalence was 11% for men and 19% for women in rural areas, and 23% and 40% in urban areas for men and women.

The systematic review by Raza et al. (2013) found only seven studies among the immigrant Pakistani community and 24 studies among the indigenous Pakistani community. They found that studies had limitations such as low participation rates and use of self-reported data. They report a higher prevalence of central obesity among women (42.2%) than among men (14.7%) (National Health Survey of Pakistan). Interestingly, differences were found along the lines of inter-ethnic groups; for example, Muhajir and Baluchis showed a higher prevalence of cardiovascular disease risk factors when compared to other ethnicities in the indigenous Pakistani population.

Health behaviour in Pakistan

Nisar et al. (2008), in her sample of university medical students, found that an unhealthy lifestyle and poor dietary habits were highly prevalent in the overweight study population.

Aslam et al. (2004) looked at the cardiovascular health behaviour of medical students in Karachi, Pakistan. They found that 8% smoked, 9% were overweight, 33% had a family history of coronary artery disease, 32% regulated dietary fat intake and 28% exercised regularly. As regards to developing cardiovascular disease in the future, 62% showed concern but only 54% of the population had adopted preventative practices. Amongst others, poor screening practices and lack of awareness were identified as barriers to changing health behaviours.

Qidwai et al. (2003) found, in their sample of 393 patients, a preference for consumption of fats/oils, sweets, spicy foods, salts and cola drinks. Furthermore, 19% of the sample reported sleeping less than six hours per day, and water consumption of less than one litre was reported by 21% of the sample.

Health information

Ludwig et al. (2011), in their study of social and cultural construction of obesity among Pakistani Muslim women in North West England, found that 55 participants lacked the motivation to address weight gain and were unsure how to do so. There was also a lack of awareness of the link between weight gain and type 2 diabetes.

Physical activity

Regular physical activity plays an important role in improving and maintaining one's health, especially as one ages. They found that, although many older American people are aware of the benefits of exercising regularly, many do not engage in physical activity as recommended by health professionals (Costello et al., 2011). This suggests that, although health messages are reaching individuals, the problem lies around changing behaviours that will increase their participation in physical activity.

A study of patterns of physical activity and the relationship with risk markers for cardiovascular disease in South Asian and European adults in a UK population by Hayes et al. (2002) found Europeans were more physically active than Indians, Pakistanis or Bangladeshis. On the physical activity index, they found 52% of European men did not meet current guidelines for participation in physical activity compared with 71% of Indians, 88% of Pakistanis and 87% of Bangladeshis. Similar findings are reported for women. Further, the level of physical activity was inversely correlated with body mass index, waist measurement, systolic blood pressure, blood glucose and insulin in all ethnic groups, but did not correlate with high-density lipoprotein (HDL) cholesterol.

Sajwani et al. (2009) compared the differences in knowledge and practices regarding healthy lifestyle among medical and non-medical students along with assessment of any perceived barriers. They found that 'lack of time' was cited as the most important reason for skipping meals and as a barrier to exercising regularly among both people

Sedentary lifestyle

Research has shown that a sedentary lifestyle, a diet in saturated fat and cholesterol, smoking and stress, as well as mortality from cardiovascular disease, varies considerably among the ethnic and cultural adult population (Savage and Harlan, 1991). Similarly, Dodani et al. (2004) in their study of risk factors of coronary heart disease in Karachi found that a very high prevalence of sedentary lifestyle, despite a high literacy rate and awareness regarding CHD risk factors, was low.

Smoking

Smoking is the single most important avoidable cause of premature morbidity and mortality in the world and it is major health problem in Pakistan (Khuwaja and Kadir, 2004; see also Gilani and Leon, 2013).

Almost a fifth of the world's tobacco is consumed in smokeless form and its consumption is common in South Asia and there are many varieties of smokeless tobacco (SLT) (Khan et al., 2014). Tobacco is chewed enormously in Pakistan; for example, paan is a kind of piper betel leaf that contains areca nut, lime, condiment and sweeteners. Another form of common SLT products used in Pakistan is naswar and has been linked to oral and oesophageal cancer (Zakiullah, 2012; see also Bile et al., 2010).

There are regional differences in Pakistan; for example, Bile et al. (2010) found that Urdu-speaking communities had a proportionately higher rate of oropharyngeal cancer (20.4%) followed by Balochis (19.9%), Sindhis (16.8%), Punjabis (11.7%) and Pashtuns (9.6%).

Alam (1998) looked at the prevalence and pattern of smoking in Pakistan from their sample of 9,441 participants, in which a total of 21.6% (36% males and 9% females) were smokers. They found that 20.7% of men in urban areas and 22% of men in rural areas were smokers. Males were more likely to be smokers than females. Further, the number of smokers who used cigarette/beedi were more likely to be males than females, while chillum/huqqa smokers were more likely to be females than males. Socioeconomic differences were found among both males and females; illiterate, and married people who had poor general health were more likely to smoke.

Similarly, a later study by Ali et al. (2008) in Sindh, Pakistan found that 10% of women were smokers and 42% of the 18-24 age group were smokers. The prevalence of smoking increased with age and income and was highest among participants aged 44 and with incomes of more than PKR 4000.

Khuwaja and Kadir's (2004) study of smoking among adult males in an urban community of Karachi found that the majority of smokers (55%) started smoking below the age of 25. Further, 42% of the adult male smokers used tobacco in other forms as well, while 58% of smokers smoked to relieve anger and frustration, or because of friends and peer pressure.

Smokeless tobacco (SLT) is linked to poor oral health and cancers. Ali et al.'s (2009) study into the usage among adult patients who visited family practices in Karachi found that, overall, 52.4% had used SLT at least in one form and more males than females were using SLT than females. They found most of the samples had started using SLT before the age of 15, 40.2% had started using SLT because of media advertisements and 30.8% due to friends/peer pressure.

Health outcomes: Cardiovascular disease

Cardiovascular disease (CVD) has become a major clinical and public health problem (Ramaraj, 2008). Stroke is the most common neurological cause of morbidity and mortality all over the world, being the third leading cause of death (Khan, 2009).

In the developed countries, Zaninotto et al. (2007), using data from the Health Surveys for England, showed that CVD was relatively more common among South Asian populations, with Black Caribbean and South Asian populations having a considerably higher chance of developing diabetes. In particular, migrant South Asian populations residing in the West have one of the highest rates of CAD in the world (Jafar et al., 2005; see also Jafar et al., 2003; Jafar et al., 2008).

Despite improvements in cardiovascular outcomes, coronary heart disease continues to be the major cause of death worldwide. South Asians have an increased risk of atherosclerosis and have the highest mortality rates from coronary artery disease (CAD) than any other ethnic group. The increased susceptibility of South Asians to CAD cannot be explained entirely by conventional risk factors alone. Other factors are involved, for example genetic disposition and high prevalence of the metabolic syndrome and type-2 diabetes. CAD is more severe, extensive and malignant among South Asians. Further, it is often unsuspected and associated with adverse outcomes requiring a more aggressive management strategy (Bainey et al., 2009).

Cardiovascular disease in Pakistan

South Asian countries, India, Pakistan, Sri Lanka, Bangladesh and Nepal not only represent a quarter of the world's population, but also contribute to the highest proportion of CVD burden when compared with any other regions globally (Ramaraj, 2008).

South Asians have a higher than average risk of CHD, although the reasons for this are unclear, but physical inactivity and/or poor responsiveness to exercise may play a role (Arjunan, 2013). The high prevalence of insulin resistance and type 2 diabetes mellitus in South Asians may be a major cause for their evaluated vascular risk (Tziomalos, 2008).

Dodani et al.'s (2004) study examined the prevalence and awareness of risk factors and risk behaviours of coronary heart disease (CHD) in the lower middle class residing in urban localities of Karachi. They found that the prevalence of hypertension (38.5%), high cholesterol (10.7%) and diabetes (9.1%) and 52.2% of the sample was overweight or obese; 64.8% never exercised and 11.9% had two or more major risk factors of CHD.

The recent study by Nadeem et al. (2013) examining the risk factors for coronary heart disease in patients below 45 years of age found, in their sample of 109 patients, cigarette smoking (46%), hypertension (37%), dyslipidemia (33%), diabetes mellitus (18%) and above normal BMI (63.3%) are the most common risk factors (see also Rafique and Khuwaja, 2003).

Jafar (2006) found that women in Pakistan have an increased burden of clinical cardiovascular risk factors than men. Modifiable factors including obesity and saturated fat intake are associated with increased prevalence of CVD risk factors, hence the urgent need to target this group in CVD prevention.

Stroke

Stroke is a major public health problem in developing countries of South Asia (Farooq et al., 2009). South Asia has 20 per cent of the world's population and has one of the highest burdens of cardiovascular disease in the world. With an aging population there is the very likely increase in the incidence of stroke in developing countries like Pakistan (Hashmi et al., 2013). Limited data available from Pakistan indicate that stroke epidemiology differs between Pakistan and Western populations. However, they highlight that, in Pakistan, stroke occurs at a younger age, particularly among women, and there is a higher proportion of haemorrhagic strokes (Farooq et al., 2009).

Stroke rates in middle-aged people are five to ten times higher in Pakistan compared with the United Kingdom or United States. There has been limited progress in Pakistan due to a number of reasons, including poor awareness on the part of patients and general physicians on stroke symptomatology, management of stroke risk factors and limited knowledge of physicians on the role of rehabilitation and its different aspects in the management of post-stroke disability (Hashmi et al., 2013).

Diabetes

There is a strong association between diabetes and obesity (Ali et al., 2014).

Type 2 diabetes is highly prevalent among people of a Pakistani background (Mygind, 2013). In addition, Nisar et al. (2008) found that type 2 diabetes mellitus was common among parents and grandparents, making the student population prone to diabetes.

Masood and Afzal (2013) examined the prevalence of diabetes mellitus and its chronic complications along with co-morbidities contributing to atherosclerosis in the diabetic population of Mirpur, Azad Kashmir, with an initial sample of 3,602 patients. Of them, 318 were diabetics, the prevalence rate being 8.83%. Of the 318 patient study subjects, 24 (7.3%) had a history of stroke, 4 (1.3%) had a history of transient ischaemic attack, 17 (5.3%) had history of myocardial infarction, and 27 (8.5%) had a history of angina. Foot ulcers were present in 22 (6.9%) and 3 (.9%) had an amputation. Co-morbid hypertension was found in 153 (48.1%) of cases, whereas co-morbid hypercholesterolaemia was found in 66 (20.8%) and 56.9% had a family history of diabetes mellitus (see Fawwad et al., 2013).

There is also a strong indication that obesity increases over time. Fawwad et al.'s (2013) study into the changing patterns of diabetes in young adults from the rural area of Baluchistan, conducted at two time points in 2002 and 2009, found that obesity had increased significantly from 20 (10.15%) in young adults in the year 2002 to 64 (27.82%).

Diabetes and religious practice

Studies indicate that many Muslims with type 2 diabetes fast during the month of Ramadan but without adequate counselling on how to adjust their medicines. Although Islam allows ill people to refrain from fasting during Ramadan, the study by Mygind et al. (2013) found that all the participants in their sample had fasted during Ramadan and had type 2 diabetes. The study showed that they adapted their use of medicines in different ways, for example changing the time of intake or by skipping morning medicines. Respondents perceived a feeling of improvement in well-being, including physiological, social and religious aspects. However, major changes in dietary habits, daily physical activities and sleeping patterns during Ramadan have significant impact on glycaemic control, lipid profile, weight and dietary intake (Hui and Devendra, 2010). Interestingly, health professionals were rarely included in the decision-making process; instead, it was friends and relatives, especially in the case of type 2 diabetes, that were considered important to the decision-making process (Mygind et al., 2013).

Hypertension

Akatsu and Aslam (1996) looked at the prevalence of hypertension and obesity among 151 women over the age of 25 in low income/underprivileged areas of Karachi, Pakistan. They found that 42% were overweight and 8% were obese. Most of the overweight/obese females had an upper body type obesity, which is an increased cardiovascular risk. The suggested interventions included diet education and weight monitoring by the community health workers.

Jafar et al. (2003), in their ethnic subgroup differences in hypertension in Pakistan, found that a threefold difference in prevalence of hypertension exists between people of South Asian descent. Interestingly, unlike the rural or urban areas, the difference cannot be accounted for by measured risk factors. Fawwad et al. (2013), in their study of young adults in Baluchistan, found an increase in hypertension increased from 13 (6.6%) in 2002 to 17 (7.39%) in their 2009 sample. Gender differences were highlighted by Ali et al. (2014), who found that females had relatively higher BMI and hypertension was more prevalent in obese diabetic patients.

Cancer

Marlow et al. (2012) explored awareness of cancer risk factors in ethnic minority men and women in England. The most commonly cited cancer risk factors were smoking (55%), diet (20%), genetics (20%) and lifestyle (17%). On average, participants were able to name cancer risk factors (91% of respondents) and cited 2.13 factors. The awareness of risk factors (particularly diet and exercise) was lower in this sample than other representative samples in the UK. They suggested interventions aimed at raising risk factors are likely to prove beneficial to ethnic minority groups. Fawwad et al. (2013) in their study of young adults in Baluchistan found that smoking increased from 8 (4.06%) in 2002 to 49 (21.3%) in 2009.

Access to services

Studies have shown that South Asians face barriers when accessing health services. Deaths from long-term health conditions (LTHCs) are set to escalate rapidly worldwide over the coming decade. Many people from South Asian backgrounds in the UK face an increased risk of such conditions as a result of severe health inequalities compared with the majority of the population (Hipwell et al., 2008). Studies examining the utilisation of hospital services by South Asian patients in the UK have consistently highlighted levels of dissatisfaction with care in relation to meeting religious and cultural needs (Vydelingum, 2000; Lindesay et al., 1997).

Language

Communication is the greatest barrier in health care provision for people of non-English speaking backgrounds (Lee et al., 2005). For example, Phul et al. (2003) found that, as a result, they have insufficient knowledge about the range of health services available and it is difficult to obtain adequate access to healthcare and health information.

There is a dearth of literature that has reported associations between low literacy and less appropriate access to healthcare services (Easton et al., 2013; Brooks et al., 2000). For example, those who arrive as refugees have experienced poor health and limited access to healthcare services (Riggs et al., 2012). Blignault et al. (2008), in their qualitative study of barriers to mental health services utilisation among migrants, found that, although Chinese-language speakers comprise the largest non-English speaking population in Australia, they have the lowest rates of mental health utilisation. They conclude that mental health services must become more culturally competent in their attempts to engage the target group. The study by Houston and Cowley (2003) showed, through using one vignette, the practical and difficult issues when a formal system is used to assess needs in clients who do not speak English as a first language.

Cultural and language differences between host country and migrants from non-English speaking backgrounds can affect the use of health services (Chan and Quine, 1997). Similarly, the study by Watt et al. (1993) conducted in Hull, UK found that language difficulties is a major barrier in seeking health services. Further, poor communication and attitudes of staff act as an underlying problem between health professionals and service users (Davies and Bath, 2001). ‘Stereotyping’ was negatively affecting the health care received by Asian women in Great Britain (Bowler, 1993). Similarly, Lowe et al. (2007) highlighted considerable institutional barriers to accessing services.

To alleviate and to be inclusive, Yeowell (2010) suggests that a culturally competent health care needs to be provided where health professionals have some understanding of the culture of their local community, thus enabling them to incorporate the patient's culture into their management. However, Hipwell et al. (2008) highlight the complexity of implementing both culturally-integrated and ethnically-specific public health interventions. Riggs et al. (2012) suggest that there is a need for a systems-oriented approach to improve service utilisation. There is a responsibility to provide equitable services irrespective of a patient's linguistic background, which proactively seek to overcome the disadvantage experienced by minority patients (Gerrish, 2001).

Interpreters

The use of interpreters may provide a solution to helping non-English speakers gain access to health services. However, there are a number of cultural and social concerns; for example, Richters and Khoei (2008) found that females are reluctant to use interpreters because of the lack of faith in their right to confidentiality. Similarly, Wellock (2010) found that female non-English speakers would not ordinarily divulge information to interpreters or relatives because of confidentiality and gossiping in the community.

Dunckley et al. (2003) suggest that translations into appropriate languages can overcome communication barriers and overlook the need for family members to act as interpreters for patients. For some, the problem is one of illiteracy, as is the case in Pakistan. The national language of Pakistan is Urdu and, although Urdu is spoken widely, given the illiteracy levels, much of the population is unable to read or write in Urdu. A further concern is that interpreters who lack appropriate training will fail to interpret accurately (Laws et al., 2004).

Ali et al. (2008) found that, among adult women in a rural district of Sindh, Pakistan, approximately 71% of women were illiterate and 44% of women between the ages of 18 and 24 were illiterate.

CHAPTER THREE

THE PAKISTANIS IN MIRPUR

When we think of 'Mirpur' we think of British Pakistanis who immigrated to the UK and, in particular, to Bradford (as well as other towns and cities such as Birmingham, Manchester and parts of London). Mirpur is a major city in Pakistan with historical links to Bradford. Some authors have labelled the city as 'Bradistan', an affectionate term to describe the existing and continued influence of Pakistan upon its residents in Bradford; examples of these are through maintaining close ties to relatives and through arranged marriages.

There has been an established historical link between Mirpur and Bradford since the late 1950s and early 1960s with the immigration of thousands of Pakistanis arriving from Mirpur and settling in Bradford to seek better financial opportunities. The continued link is seen through the 'keeping up of the traditions', for example the sending of remittances, arranged marriages and the regular visits to see relatives left behind. This continuation of traditions (particularly for older people) is important to maintaining close ties.

History of Pakistanis (Din, 2006)

After the separation of East and West Pakistan (later Bangladesh and Pakistan) in 1947 from India, Mirpur became one of the three districts of Azad 'Free' Kashmir (Rose et al., 1969) and the majority of Pakistanis came from this region (Shaw, 2001). The majority of Pakistanis who settled in the UK resided in Bradford and Birmingham (Allen, 1971; Taylor, 1976; Dahya, 1972-77; Shaw, 1988, 2000; Werbner, 1990).

There were several major reasons for the partition. Robinson (1993) argues that Muslim separatism was fostered both by the political needs of the British and by those of Hindus and Muslims. According to Robinson, this was important because the religious differences that separated Muslims from the Hindus were fundamental. For example, Hindus worshipped idols, whereas Muslims abhorred them. Hindus had many gods, the Muslims have one God. This created tension between the Hindu population and the Muslims, who were in the minority. In addition, Muslims feared that the Hindu majority would not only interfere with Muslim religious practices, such as cow-sacrifices, but also religious differences would lead to discrimination against them in wider secular fields such as in education and in employment (Robinson, 1993; Brown and Foot, 1994).

After independence, Pakistan went through a number of social changes. This included, for example, the spread of primary school education, especially Islamic education and ideas of nationalism with reference to Kashmir. However, progress on the whole was slow, and unemployment was high (Rose et al., 1969; Taylor, 1976; Holmes, 1991). An illustration of poverty in Pakistan in the 1940s and the 1950s was the low literacy rate, as well as the poor provision of schooling (Braham, 1992). Due to high levels of poverty within the district of Mirpur, only a small number of young children entered secondary schooling and less than half stayed on at the age of 15. Thus, it is not surprising that the majority of the immigrants who came to Britain were illiterate (Khan, 1979; Kannon, 1978). It was estimated that unemployment was 7.4 million at the end of 1964 (Economist Intelligence Unit, 1966). According to the speech made by the President of Pakistan, Ayub Khan, at the time the per capita income was only £30 per annum (Rose et al., 1969).

To increase electrical output, the Pakistani government made a decision to build the world's largest hydroelectric earth dam at Mangla, which was constructed during the late 1950s and the early 1960s. As a result, it submerged 250 villages in the district of Mirpur and displaced approximately 100,000 people. As a result of the dam, a new Mirpur city emerged at the side of the lake, which replaced the old Mirpur town. Other displaced families were allocated land in the state of Punjab (Taylor, 1976; Holmes, 1991; Anwar, 1998).

Most families living in Mirpur were connected with the land; the majority were small peasant farmers or landless labourers (Taylor, 1976; Lewis, 1994). Dahya found that two-thirds of the 200 respondents interviewed had been farming their family land prior to migration. Furthermore, nearly half had been in the Armed Forces or had served in the Merchant Navy.

Family life

The village household is often three-generational, comprising of grandparent(s), married son(s), their wives(s) and children and unmarried son(s) and daughter(s). Property is communally owned, whether the source of this is through work, land or wage labour, and decisions are communally made. The final decision rests with the head of the family, the eldest male, and authority is allocated according to gender and age (Khan, 1979). It is important to bear in mind that the izzat of the family is crucial for parents and biraderi elders.

Beyond the household, there are biraderi members (kin groups) whose members claim descent in a paternal line from a common male ancestor. Raza (1993) argued that, in village society, the individual forms part of a complex network of rights and obligations, which extend outwards from his/her immediate family to that of kin and fellow villagers. He defined biraderi as, ‘it includes all men who can trace their relationship to a common ancestor, no matter how remote’.

Individualism and independence, so revered by the West, appears selfish to Pakistanis, who expect and value dependency and loyalty to kin members and kin groups. Within the Pakistani family, individual rights are dictated by age, sex and the order of birth. One of the main characteristics of village life is that everyone knows each other: close friends are classified as ‘brothers’ and ‘sisters’. This network of friends and family also ensures conformity and deviants are ‘pulled back’ into line by the community (Khan, 1979; Rapoport et al., 1982). The family is the vehicle for conveying the group norms to ensure its survival is sustained by a religious ethos, and it is the religious element that gives these norms the strength and enforces the values of the biraderi (Basit, 1997). Individualism fostered by the white culture is almost unknown to people from rural Pakistan, who work and live together and where individuals are expected to be loyal and respectful to fellow kin members. In cases of disobedience, social pressure is exercised on its members to conform to traditional values (Hiro, 1991). This still holds true today.

In terms of biraderi relations, Raza argued that the individual does not act on his own behalf, but his/her reputation depends upon theirs and the fulfilling of obligations ascribed to him which, as a result, keeps the family ‘bound’ together (Raza, 1993). Wilson (1978) defined izzat as ‘the sensitive and many faceted male identity which can change as the situation demands it – from family honour to self-respect and sometimes to pure male ego’ (in Adams, 1978). Ballard argued that, in its narrow sense, ‘izzat’ is a matter of male pride (Rapoport et al., 1982).

Caste

In order to understand this community, it is important to explain their belief in the caste system. Before the independence of Pakistan from India in 1947, Muslims, Hindus and Sikhs lived together in towns and villages across India, although each of these communities had their own traditions, norms and beliefs. Over a period of time, some of the traits of Hinduism and Sikhism became fused into the culture of Pakistanis/Muslims. This fusion between the Hindu and the Pakistani culture can be seen from examining marriage rituals and the practice of dowry. In Hinduism, the family of the bride must give a dowry to the groom, which can include a combination of money, gold and land (especially in Pakistan).

Singh (1959) found that, before the separation of Pakistan, Muslims, Sikhs and Hindus commonly visited one another's shrines and that many Muslim holy men had Hindu followers (Taylor, 1976). Caste plays an important part in the lives of Hindus, which determines the life chances of every individual. The highest caste in Hinduism is Brahman (Pardesh, 1994). Men born in this caste become priests and scholars and provide the spiritual leadership of their community. At the bottom of the caste hierarchy, and those deprived of caste affiliation, are the outcasts who are labelled as engaging in demeaning or polluting occupations by the society. The origins of the caste system can be dated as far back as 1500 BC to the ancient sacred writing of Rig-Veda (Skjonsberg, 1982).

Social stratification in Pakistan is based on the caste system. Unlike the Hindu system, the Pakistani caste system is not religiously based, but cultural. The highest caste in Pakistan is the Rajah or Jats, who are the landed gentry, the traditional ruling class in Pakistan. The lowest castes are Kamini, landless labourers, for example the Majaar caste, who may be shoesmiths, blacksmiths, etc. (Ranger et al., 1996). The social structure of the villages from which migrants are drawn closely parallels that of a Hindu caste system made up of a number of largely endogamous and nominally occupationally-linked descent groups (Shaw, 1994).

'The land of dreams'

Britain has a long history of white and non-white immigration to its shores. The presence of Asians in Britain can be dated back to the seventeenth century (Fryer, 1984; Visram, 1986). Indians began coming to the UK from the early part of the twentieth century as seamen (Aurora, 1976; Desai, 1963) and settled in areas such as Birmingham (Rose et al., 1969). Others, mainly white people, arrived from Europe and Eastern Europe. The numbers increased dramatically, especially after World War II. The mass migration of non-white workers started more slowly but, during the 1950s, increased substantially in the number of migrants from the West Indies. Although mass migration from India and Pakistan began from 1945, it also reached a high level from 1960 onwards (Anwar, 1995).

In reality, there were few economic reasons to encourage Pakistani men to stay in Mirpur or indeed Pakistan (Khan, 1979; Holmes, 1991; Lewis, 1994). To those who had relatives or fellow kinsmen who were already settled in the UK, unlimited opportunities proved to be an important deciding factor in chain migration. Another motive for lower-caste families to immigrate was free 'vilayati' (English) education, which could improve the status of an individual as well as that of the family, whereas lower-caste groups had always been subjugated by those higher than them and never had the opportunity to climb up the social hierarchy (Kannon, 1978).

Roger Ballard argued that the early immigrants were drawn from peasant families with limited land holdings who could use overseas earnings to redeem mortgaged land, as well as buy more to provide sisters with dowries, to build new houses and to purchase agricultural implements (Rapoport et al., 1982). This was at a cost to those living in Britain, since most of the savings were sent to those relatives still left behind. They had to do without material things such as televisions. However, not all migrants who came to Britain were small farmers. A small number of urban educated middle-class migrants also arrived in Britain in the 1960s (Braham, 1992).

Sending remittances still remains a habit which has been long-established and remains standard among many older Pakistanis. Khan (1979) found that the remittances sent to Mirpur improved both the general standard of living and also contributed towards the economy of Mirpur through investment. The early Pakistanis remitted as much as half of their earnings. It was estimated that, in 1963, £26 million was remitted, which amounted to more than the whole inland revenue of East Pakistan (Khan, 1979; Lewis, 1994). This demonstrates a dependent connection between kin in Britain and those who still remained back in Mirpur. Many large, new houses were built in the new Mirpur City with remittances sent by relatives from Britain (Lewis, 1994). This would ensure that close ties with the country of origin would continue (Khan, 1979). Most built houses to show off their wealth to biraderi, but also to non-biraderi members. This gave most a sense of satisfaction that 'they had made it'; but, at the same time, this created resentment and hostility among biraderi members.

The money sent to Pakistan was used to pay off debts and to support family and relatives. Some early successful Pakistanis living and working in Britain invested large amounts of money in Mirpur. Dahya (1973), for example, found that, in the district of Jehlum, Pakistani migrants had built a cinema, petrol station and flats (Khan, 1979).

Diet after Independence

The diet, especially after Independence, was pretty ‘simple’ (due to lack of affordability) compared to the present day. The ‘basics’, including roti and curry (vegetable, lentils), were served every day and meat was served once a week or on special occasions such as on Eid or when the family was entertaining special visitors, often those from overseas, for example from the UK. Pakistanis with all their ingenuity to survive made the most of staple ingredients; for example, potatoes are a versatile vegetable and, when cooked as a curry with a few spices, make it appetizing for hungry mouths. Most vegetables such as potatoes, carrots, aubergines and okra were grown at home in the vegetable patch, which allowed the family to survive, but flour had to be purchased from the bazaar (market). All the money earned by family members was spent on buying flour. In fact, the wealth of the Pakistani family was judged by the amount of flour they had in the home (it was gold dust).

Other staple foods such as milk were luxury products. If the resources allowed, then the family would purchase a small quantity of milk from a neighbour who could afford and keep a cow. Most often, the family would have black tea and, again, if resources allowed, they would have tea with cardamom seeds which would give black tea some flavour. Tea in Pakistan is made differently to the Western version. Most Pakistanis make tea with milk (few add a small quantity of water); it is a filling drink that, even on its own, could keep a stomach filled until lunchtime. Another rarity was sugar, which was expensive and only those with good incomes could afford to have it in Pakistan.

CHAPTER FOUR

RESEARCHING THE BRITISH PAKISTANIS

Introduction

This chapter examines research methods helping researchers to think about the way in which they go about collecting fieldwork data. Firstly, to understand minority communities (in this case, the Pakistanis). Secondly, the appropriate methods that help them to reach the desired goals and outcomes of data collection. How you reach the decision as regards to the methods that will be employed will depend upon one's epistemological background embedded in the theoretical perspective in the methodology.

Increasing participation of South Asians in research studies

The increasing culturally diverse groups in the UK have meant that barriers such as language need to be addressed. The recruitment of respondents with English as a second language to research studies is essential if their unique and valid perspective is to be acknowledged (Marshall and While, 1994).

Families from socioeconomically deprived and ethnic minority groups are less likely to participate in health services research and those who are likely to take part in research are more likely to be white British and from higher socioeconomic groups (Rahi et al., 2004).

The failure to include and/or identify subgroups of the population can undermine the value of research. This can have an impact on needs assessments and service delivery (Yildiz and Barnett, 2011).

Including participants from diverse backgrounds has a number of advantages for participants; for example, the evaluation by Fudge et al. (2007) on involving older people in health research focussed on the impact on participants and highlighted a number of benefits to participants, including increased knowledge, awareness and confidence, meeting others in a similar situation, as well as empowering older people in health research.

In their 2004 study, Hussain-Gambles highlighted a number of effective strategies that can be used to recruit South Asians to clinical trials, including ensuring the eligibility criteria are set as wide as possible, determining the most effective mass media to use in study promotion, and the recruitment and consulting of representative community members to provide assistance in the study. The latter involves asking the help of community leaders and elders to help in recruitment and publicising the study. Although elders would generally like to help researchers, they need to ensure that elders communicate the correct information to potential participants. However, the pitfall is when the researcher does not speak the language of the elder's community and there is no way of checking whether the study information is correctly translated to participants.

The later study by Hussain-Gambles et al. (2006) found that, although there was no antipathy amongst South Asians to the concept of clinical trials, a number of factors were highlighted that may act as a barrier, including age, language, social class, feeling of not belonging/mistrust and culture and religion. As a result, South Asians may be systematically excluded from trials because of the increased cost and time associated with their inclusion, particularly in relation to language barrier. They report that under-representation might also be due to passive exclusion associated with cultural stereotypes, and that the existence of an exclusionary health care culture continues to affect equity and access for people of a non-English speaking background (Blackford and Street, 2002).

The study by Homer (2000) highlighted that randomised controlled trials exclude women who do not speak English, or are designed in such a way that cultural diversity is not facilitated. This can lead to a sample that is unrepresentative of the population from which it was drawn or to which it will be applied. Homer points out that culturally diverse representation can be achieved through employing a number of strategies, including utilising health-care interpreters, ensuring materials are translated into common community languages and engaging the local community. This should ensure that the sample in a randomised controlled trial is culturally and linguistically diverse.

Similarly, changing population demographics and immigration patterns have resulted in increasing numbers of Canadians speaking a language other French or English. The inclusion of non-English speaking groups is important if disparities in access and use of preventive health care services are to addressed (Thomson and Hoffman-Goetz, 2011).

In the study by Plumridge et al. (2013), which looked at the under-representation of minority ethnic groups in cardiovascular research, it found that few participants had any understanding of the objectives and nature of research. If this is explained to potential participants, many would describe altruistic reasons for why they would participate in research in the future. The willingness to take part in research as long as participants are approached directly and the reasons for research and potential benefits are explained to them. It is important to build a rapport with participants, but this involves time commitment on the part of the researcher and spending time at the places of recruitment is important.

Researchers face challenges when obtaining consent from participants since the majority of the general population has limited or no familiarity with research studies. This is further problematic when obtaining consent from individuals with low literacy levels and those who speak languages other than English (Cortes et al., 2010). One case in point is that the national language of Pakistan is Urdu; however, there are many dialects which are spoken locally. For example, many Pakistanis living in Bradford speak Mirpuri, Punjabi or Kashmiri and these dialects have no written equivalent, thus information sheets and consent forms cannot be devised. There are alternatives, for example having verbal consents instead of written consents, and the Information Sheets can also be verbally translated. However, one main disadvantage is that, in many cases, participants like to read the information at their leisure and then decide whether they would like to participate. Another problem is that, even if researchers speak the same dialect, they will most likely translate information differently; there is also the possibility of 'glazing' over certain information. Other areas of concern in health research is that medical terms are difficult to translate into a dialect, especially if one is recruiting patients for clinical trials.

A study by Hunt and Bhopal (2004) highlighted a number of potential pitfalls where instruments that are designed for English speakers are simply translated into ethnic minority languages, where measurement error can result from inadequate translation procedures, inappropriate content, insensitivity of items and the failure of researchers to make themselves familiar with cultural norms and beliefs. The latter is paramount in understanding minority ethnic communities, and being aware of such issues allows the research to be transmitted in culturally acceptable terms. The point to remember is that 'one size does not fit all'. These issues should be dealt with at the exploratory or pilot stage and, with careful planning, many of the barriers can be overcome.

The study by Hanna et al. (2012) highlights some of the pitfalls of translating material into community languages. Participants were asked to elaborate on their understanding of the question and meaning of keywords or phrases. For example, the translation for 'chest' was interpreted by some Pakistani and Chinese women to mean 'breasts', and 'walking up the hill' was translated in Chinese as 'walking the hill', an interpretation pertaining to walking downhill.

Using interpreters for research purposes

For purposes of research, Simon et al. (2006) show that language interpreters mediate a growing number of health care communication events, including the informed consent process which underlies the ethical conduct of clinical research. They highlight the concern around the accuracy of the interpretation, for example the concept of 'randomisation', often poorly communicated and interpreted, and that clinicians need to use less technical language and shorter sentences and to be more 'process driven'. The type of methods used by the research study are important; for example, Twinn (1997) suggests there can be particular problems in using translations in phenomenological research designs.

Fieldwork: arranging interviews (Din, 2008)

The interview is a fluid process allowing the participants the opportunity to ask questions or take a break from answering questions. It also allows participants enough flexibility to change the focus of the interview in order to raise issues or change direction; the researcher should adapt the questions accordingly. To allow for this, there were no pre-set questions, nor was a traditional topic guide written. Most interviews begin with pre-set questions to be discussed with participants, which do not allow or have limited opportunity to allow a participant to steer away from specific questions. These questions are answered in a question-answer session; the participant is guided through the topic guide or an interview schedule. This can lack fluidity.

Research questions develop as the study progresses and may mean that the direction of the research changes. It is practically impossible to predict what participants will say or whether they will raise issues of importance. Research can be preset in other ways. Often, the cohort and the sample ranges are decided before the data collection phase. Practically, it may be difficult to get that precise number of participants recruited for the study, or even interested in taking part. More seriously, there is the issue of reliability; it is difficult to predict that *x* number of interviews will provide a sufficient consistency in the data to stop interviewing, or indeed it may be necessary to conduct further interviews.

For most, the easiest or most simple way of recruiting individuals to take part in research is to send a letter to their home or contact them through a community centre, and this is often used when recruiting older people for research. Contacting people at home can raise questions about ethics, even when interviewing parents. In the case of the Pakistani community, one-to-one interviews are difficult to arrange and hold, given the cultural norms. For example, if one were to arrange an interview with a mother, it would be expected that she will be joined by her husband in the same room; he may also contribute to the interview or perhaps even 'take over' the conversation. Relatives who are visiting can also take part for these reasons. The researcher and the research can be a topical point of discussion, as well as inquisitive questions such as: Who is he/she? Where is he/she from? What did he/she want to talk about? They can be questions that the interviewee may answer once the researcher has left.

It should be noted that it can often be difficult for the researcher to ask people to leave the room because he/she is an 'invited guest' (Din, 2006). In any case, it should not be left to the interviewee to make the decision. This raises serious issues of confidentiality. For this reason, keeping conversations private can be more difficult if the interview is conducted at home. Remembering cultural norms and practices ensures the interview runs smoothly and allows participants to feel comfortable. Taking this into account, obtaining informed consent is also an issue when the interviewee is joined by member(s) of the family/relatives. This is particularly correct in Pakistan where relatives live in joint households; for example, it is not uncommon to find the husband, wife, children, grandparents and married siblings living in the same household. For research purposes, it is practically impossible to conduct any type of interview without other members of the household being present.

There are a number of questions to be considered before, during and after the completion of the project. For example, how will participants be contacted? (by letter, telephone or in person?); is the information on the research in an appropriate language? (researchers may wish to consider making information available on an audio tape, which will allow non-English speakers to listen to the information as opposed to relying on family members/relatives to translate the written information); the gender of the researcher; the location of the interviews; will the information be tape recorded? (researchers can find there is a general reluctance for participants to be recorded); how will the final report be disseminated? This is often done through formal channels, for example at a university or in community centres. However, most attendees are often male and few females are likely to attend, so researchers need to ensure appropriate ways of disseminating the findings depending on the type of project. Although this adds to the overall budget of the research, final reports should be made available in different languages of the participants and also on audio tape for those who are unable to read.

The researcher needs to do his/her ‘homework’ before arranging the interview. The researcher also has to be an active participant. Arranging interviews away from the place of work and in the preferred ‘home environment’ of the participant should be used as an opportunity to get to know the community (especially if the researcher is from outside the district/community). So, instead of parking outside the participant’s house waiting for the exact time to knock on the door, it is advisable to park elsewhere and take a walk around the streets, go into shops or visit a cafe for lunch.

If the opportunity arises to speak to the locals, quite often older men are found talking outside the mosque or shops. It is a chance to ask questions and get to know the local people and the communities they are part of. Young people can often be seen playing football or cricket in the local fields and the researcher can often be invited to join in. If the interviews are conducted during the summer vacation, voluntary organisations often arrange play days or theme days in local play areas where young people and families are invited to join in. This is a way of bringing local people together and an opportunity to get to know people from different backgrounds.

It is important for the researcher to know what is going on in the local community. This is obviously a longer process than simply conducting the interview, but it does allow the researcher to place the participant in the context of his/her community. This is another criticism by participants that, on occasions, they find the researcher is totally unfamiliar with the local surroundings, such as the location of the mosque, school, centres or college. These are quoted because they are important to the participants. It also helps researchers to actively participate (given the circumstances) and to build a broader picture of the local community.

Knowing the cultural practices of the participants is essential in building rapport between the researcher and those being researched and this can only be done if researchers know the community. This can also help to access ‘hard to reach’ communities, for example females (e.g. those from overseas who marry someone from the UK).

Knowing how to conduct oneself and the formalities before and after the interview is essential but is often overlooked. For example, the researcher should ensure that the interview is not arranged during Namaz (Prayer) or Jumma (Friday) prayer times or during the month of Ramadan

(Fasting). Upon entering the house or room (e.g. in a community centre), the researcher must remember to remove their shoes or at least offer to do so as a polite gesture. Upon entering the room, the researcher should shake hands, beginning with the eldest male member first. If there are females present, a ‘salaam’ (greetings) is sufficient and they must remember to sit near the men. It is unsuitable for a male researcher to shake hands with a female or to refuse tea/refreshments when offered (even if not required). Hospitality is an integral part of the interview. At times, the 45-minute interview can last three hours.

It is common before the more formal interview for participants to ask questions of the researcher, including personal details such as one’s age, marital status, number and age of children, names of parents, names of relatives, one’s origin in Pakistani, place of residency and occupation. This allows the participant to understand the researcher and where he/she is from. It also ‘breaks the ice’. However, those from outside the community may think such questions are too personal to be answered. It is also common at the end of the interview for the participant to ask questions or ask for help on issues totally unrelated to the interview. These can include completing paperwork or help with making telephone calls to a GP’s surgery, to the school or other organisation. It is expected that the researcher is in a position to help and will do so, especially in UK-based research.

One should bear in mind that Pakistani females, both young and old, are less likely to attend community centres because such ‘public centres’ are seen as male spaces. Culturally or traditionally, it is inappropriate for women to mix with men in communal places. This is not necessarily a reflection on centres that have done considerable amounts of work trying to attract women and the less represented groups. This is particularly relevant to the situation in Pakistan, where women rarely venture outside of the house without being escorted.

Practical tips and advice

This chapter provides helpful ‘tips and pointers’ to researchers when they recruit participants from a minority ethnic community setting, in this case the Pakistanis. Many of the examples provided in this chapter are from personal research experience on the strategies that the author has used and which have worked well, while others are reflections and pointers to steer researchers in the right direction.

As a researcher, I would be stating the obvious when I say that data collection/fieldwork is often an ‘individual activity’ having tight recruitment periods which one needs to meet. The project relies on researchers to obtain a set number of participants within a certain time period. This is closely monitored by the senior research team; questions such as 'how is the recruitment going?' are often echoed in staff kitchens and corridors; (understandably so) it often becomes 'a numbers game', especially when the sample is large.

Some studies will have a single research assistant recruiting, while others may have half a dozen researchers recruiting on a daily basis. When I have been involved in studies that have a large recruitment team, I have considered this as a 'team effort', where everyone contributes their share; it is not an individual task. On some days, one may recruit more than a colleague whilst, on other days, they may 'chip in' more than their daily total.

Keeping 'each other going' through the recruitment period is essential (partly because one's job depends upon it!) but for the fact one wants to prove they can be successful recruiters (and a team). If I compare it to a successful football team, working in a team requires a 'team effort', where everyone is rooting for the same outcome, namely a win; morale is in abundance and effort readily forthcoming. Every member of the team 'chips in', from making sure the site file is in order to having an adequate number of paper questionnaires, from making sure consent forms are correctly completed to keeping a daily log of those successfully recruited.

Research method books often ignore the fact that this can be a stressful period for (junior) fieldworkers, who are out recruiting every day, often without a break. Thoughtful senior researchers will allow for office days or recruitment-free days for field researchers. For most, it is a well-deserved break, but also a time to reflect; for example, it is an opportunity to sit back and think of things that have been enhancing recruitment, strategies that are working well, but also if recruitment is going slow then there is the need to be aware of things that have been acting as 'barriers' to recruitment. The former requires more of the same, but the latter may require a change in strategy and an opportunity to do something different. The 'free days' can be spent developing 'a plan' to overcome (hopefully) a temporary difficulty and allows one to speak to senior colleagues.

However, it is not only the fieldworkers who may be feeling under stress, but senior research and chief investigators can also be feeling 'nervy' and are often under the same pressures to make sure the study is developed on time (and within budget). Although senior researchers will be based in the office, they plan a carefully planned strategy to ensure the study completes successfully. They ensure the ethics form is successfully completed, thus ensuring they get the 'go ahead' from the research ethics committee (REC), and liaise with the R and D department to make sure the study at the site goes ahead. These two take up enormous amounts of time, especially if the forms need to be sent back for further clarification, even if they require a 'chair's action', but also if an 'amendment' needs to be put in.

They put in a substantial amount of time trying to get professionals and organisations 'on board' in order to obtain access to study sites, and all of this relies on careful planning. Often, months of preparation are spent dealing with professionals at different levels to ensure that they can recruit from the study sites, that access is allowed during recruitment and that it will run smoothly. From experience, there is 'a lot of running around' chasing professionals in order to set up meetings using a range of communication methods, for example initially making contact by e-mail and then following up with a telephone call.

The pressure is on researchers, often chasing key individuals on a daily or weekly basis. At times, it can take several weeks to meet a key individual, as annual leave, training and sickness can play a part in this delay. Whilst other times professionals do not wish to 'add to their workload', and irrespective of how many times the senior researcher may get in touch with them, their request will fail. Essentially, there is little to be gained by becoming involved in the research study (unless there is interest on the part of the researcher), otherwise it is 'free' activity but one which will inevitably require a certain amount of time and effort on the part of the professional. For this reason, it can be difficult for the researcher to have the right professionals on board and the researcher may well need to look for alternatives.

Successful studies need representative samples, and diversity is paramount which takes into account age, gender, ethnicity and socioeconomic backgrounds of participants. Furthermore, there are a whole range of 'minority within minority groups' whose voices are sometimes not heard or are not represented adequately in research studies. Good examples of groups who may be excluded include non-English speaking participants, the elderly, and those who have a learning disability; examples within these groups include older Pakistani females, white/English elderly people and older people with a learning disability.

It is important to include all groups (insofar as it is possible) because it is also about service improvement; for example, excluding non-English speaking patients in maternity services can mean that any service improvements may be limited. Research is essentially about representing individual (or community) viewpoints, and being given the opportunity to voice their opinions and to be heard.

Many towns and cities around the UK (London, Birmingham and Manchester are good examples) have diverse and transient populations. The ‘aim’ for researchers should be to achieve a representative sample, one that will reflect the local community and thus be as inclusive as possible. On the other hand, we have the pragmatics, as the difficulty of achieving the representative sample can prove to be elusive. To do this, there needs to be the will and the desire among the senior researchers.

Getting the team right is crucial. Members of the team who are pro-active, creative and imaginative will certainly come into their own, especially when recruitment is becoming difficult and when one needs to bounce ideas. So, too, will members of the steering group who should ideally be in position to give constructive advice to researchers, for example suggesting contacts in the community that can be called for help and advice. Recruitment should be a team activity.

‘Reaching out to the communities’

There are many groups that are under-represented in research studies and, in my experience, particularly from the following: those from minority ethnic communities, especially the non-English speakers, younger people (cutting across ethnic groups), the elderly, single parent white/English females, the disabled, homeless people, those suffering from mental health issues, alcoholics and drug users. They can be considered by researchers as being a difficult to recruit group, thus researchers perhaps too easily tend to target ‘easier to reach’ groups. To recruit from the above groups requires a substantial amount of time and resources to target these groups; and, the problem is, that most research studies have not ‘costed’ this in the research grant. A good example is translation and interpreting, depending upon the study; this can amount to tens of thousands of pounds, especially if interpreters are required on a daily basis. Material such as information sheets and consent forms need to be translated into different community languages.

One of the main challenges of engaging with minority ethnic communities is working out how to make contact with individuals and local groups. For many researchers (both experienced and junior) this can be a daunting task to undertake. Although support from the senior research team will be vital, it will be the role of the research assistant/research fellow to collect fieldwork data. So, where does one begin? I would like to share my experiences here and, although there is no hard and fast rule to accessing ‘hard to reach’ and marginalised groups, there are a number of things that can be done to make the process easier, thus making it less stressful.

Gatekeepers

The appeal of having ‘elders’ or gatekeepers on board for research purposes is obvious: they can help to recruit participants to research studies. Potentially, they have access to large numbers of individuals within their own community, which seems attractive to researchers. I would like to say that gatekeepers should not be the first port of call for researchers, as existing contacts should be explored first. The researcher should talk to as many researchers and lay people as possible, which is a good first step, as well as getting to know the potential sample. Researchers sometimes ‘jump in at the deep end’ without a plan or purpose and often ‘hit a brick wall’; this can lead to demotivation and, at worse, desperation. The advice is as above: keep talking to as many different people as you possibly can, learning from their experiences as you go along.

I think researchers need to be aware of two main disadvantages when using ‘gatekeepers’ for the purposes of recruitment. Firstly, gatekeepers can sometimes ‘decide about the suitability of the research’ during the initial meeting, and certainly after reading the information sheet and other study material; as an outcome, they decide whether the research would be of benefit to their users or whether it is appropriate. If the researcher has simply ‘rushed into’ the community without any thought or planning, the gatekeeper often makes a spur of the moment decision; a simple ‘yes’ or ‘no’, without any ‘second bite at the cherry’. It is in the researcher’s interest to do this properly and carefully.

Research that is considered as being ‘unsuitable’ by Pakistani gatekeepers and one that receives a negative response includes the role of women within the Pakistani community and forced arranged marriages. Also considered unsuitable is research that may ask questions about one’s lifestyle, such as sexual behaviour, and questions that are culturally insensitive, such as alcohol consumption among young Pakistani (Muslim) men.

Further, gatekeepers have a tendency to ‘select’ participants who may reflect the general opinions of the community under research. The important test for elders is that research should lead to the benefit of researchers and the individual/community alike. The important point that researchers need to bear in mind is that there has to be a certain amount of ‘give and take’.

Gatekeepers or elders have proved vital in research studies, without which studies would have not been able to fulfil minimum recruitment numbers. One area where a researcher would need the assistance of elders is if the research requires large numbers of non-English speaking patients who have type 2 diabetes. Elders with good contacts can open doors for researchers; for example, they can distribute information sheets on behalf of researchers that can be handed down to their congregation at mosques. I should point out that an enhancer to this process is if the researcher shares the same language, religion and culture as the gatekeeper, all of which would certainly help. Ideally, what the researcher needs to do is to build a lasting relationship with the gatekeeper using their knowledge as a solid base for recruitment.

Researchers and communities

Researchers from outside of the community can find this difficult and challenging without being 'let in' by the gatekeepers. It goes without saying gatekeepers need to be shown respect and gratitude, since they would be helping researchers out of the goodness of their heart and without any payment. Not all fieldworkers will be suited to this task, as some are naturally better than others. Communication skills, as well as being polite, go a long way especially in a community where these traits are considered the bedrock of its beliefs.

Researchers should understand the etiquette as well as the 'ins and outs' of researching and recruiting participants who are from a different ethnic minority group. As mentioned above, using gatekeepers is a resource-intensive activity; senior researchers involved in the study need to ensure that fieldworkers have sufficient time 'built in' and allocated to take on this task effectively, otherwise it will prove fruitless, not because of the lack of trying but because the team did not allow sufficient time. Likewise, fieldworkers should not think of this task as being 'easy', where they will simply visit community centres and talk to gatekeepers and that they will agree without reservation; both time and effort is needed, as well as a considerable amount of imagination. This is not a 'quick fix' solution to all the problems of recruiting; therefore, ignore it at your peril! It is obvious when I state that gatekeepers are not researchers and they are not paid to help researchers.

This is why 'knowing the locality' is essential and a theme that runs throughout this book. It should be like reading the neighbourhood statistics on a local level, where statistics become alive. The message here is that, without knowing 'what's going on' and understanding the population that resides in the neighbourhood, it can become a futile exercise. Bearing in mind that 'one size does not fit all', some fieldworkers will be adequately knowledgeable about the task others will be lacking in the 'know how'.

The problem in some cases is that researchers (at all levels) do not know the locality except what they have read in academic journals without actually venturing out into the community themselves. Bradford is a good case example. Riots in Bradford in 1995 and 2001 have meant that research-funding organisations have funded a number of studies that 'examine' Bradford and its populations; researchers live outside of the district and employ community fieldworkers to do the data collection, analyse the transcripts and write up the findings in a report, some of whom rarely have ventured out of the workplace. This is often a major criticism expressed by people that researchers need to 'come out' into the community and see what is going on.

'Community researchers'

Let us assume a scenario for the senior research team members. The fieldworkers have exhausted all avenues, having contacted gatekeepers. Although it has proved useful, you are still struggling to get to the finish line and there are still more participants that need to be recruited.

A way of getting round the problem of accessing 'hard to reach' communities is employing community researchers and this is gaining in popularity. Community researchers, who are part of the same community under research, who share the same language, religion, values and norm, can have a distinct advantage. There are a number advantages to employing community researchers; for example, they will know their locality particularly well, including popular places such as community centres, libraries, GP surgeries, medical centres, places of worship and places where people congregate. These can all be useful locations to visit for the purposes of recruitment.

In essence, they have their ear to the ground. In my experience, a researcher who does not reside in the area will be unfamiliar with the surroundings and it can take a substantial amount of time and effort to get to know the local area and its populations. I think this is a lost opportunity (and a concern) as they ideally need to 'go out and about' into the neighbourhood and community to see what is going on. There are many places to meet local people at events as discussed above and time needs to be allowed to do this effectively.

Researchers need to be clear about the contribution made by community researchers; for example, would they only be involved in the fieldwork? Or would they be involved in the analysis? Or dissemination activities? Community researchers certainly can help in building an overall picture of the lives of the participants and this can feed back into the analysis. Further, their experience can be invaluable during dissemination activities; community researchers can feed the findings of the study back to participants, for example they can hold workshops or feedback sessions at community centres. Since community researchers will work with professional researchers on a daily basis, the latter are in a valuable position by which to learn about the community under research.

Although some will be experienced, I think it is a good idea for members of the research team to go out into the community with community researchers. This can allow the community researcher to get over the initial hurdle of discussing the research with participants or those in charge of community centres, and the senior will be present if questions arise that require their input. It is important to remember that fieldwork is difficult even for the most experienced of researchers (irrespective of background); some relish the challenge, while many others struggle even to make initial contacts. Perseverance and a well-planned strategy are crucial.

Community researchers can prove particularly useful in longitudinal studies running over a period of months or years, since they require effort and resilience on the part of researchers to keep participants informed and 'interested' over the duration of the research. Research is about people and individuals, and good rapport and social skills are essential criteria for all researchers. These are essentially learnt in situ, in the real world; for example, meeting and greeting Pakistani elders upon entering their house. It can be difficult to learn initially, but certainly very easy to get wrong; after all, researchers need to learn the etiquette of the community under research. They need to be careful in what they do and what they say, particularly if they are 'outsiders' and do not share the host's language, religion and culture. In these situations, often interpreters are used, but one should not presume that everything that is said is easily translatable, for example humour.

Community researchers can certainly make sense of individual lives. I remember conducting fieldwork in one inner city area, where the study was looking into the needs of disabled older people and how families cope. All the families interviewed were receiving benefits and the carers had to give up work (most were employed full-time) to look after their siblings. However, the difficulty was in describing their sense of isolation, the difficulties encountered on a daily basis, the lack of family and community support. Most of their income went into paying bills and food was seen as something of a luxury. Their financial predicament was often strained to say the least; most were on prepayment meters due to arrears and they were also behind with other essential household bills.

It can be difficult to make sense of people's lives through transcripts and without understanding the context of where people reside, and often the many daily struggles to make ends meet. The meaning of this can be lost and one that respondents strive really hard to put across to researchers. If there is a benefit to taking part in research, it is to be in a position to answer questions in a way that will tell their individual story and in their own words. Again 'one size does not fit all' as different communities may require different approaches. When asked the question, older Pakistanis enjoy talking in narrative; a question that requires a reasonably short answer may turn into a long answer. Other groups enjoy the traditional 'question and answer' method.

Getting to know the sample: Places to visit

The community forms the bedrock of family life for Pakistanis, as parents and elders still regulate day to day practices. Bradford is a good example of the complex nature of individual and community life. If we take the example of the Pakistanis in Bradford, we find they are concentrated in certain wards, for example Great Horton, Little Horton, Girlington, Heaton and Thornbury. One often finds that biraderi (kin) members live close by to one another and reliance upon fellow biraderi members is paramount to Pakistanis. Most still maintain the idea that family is the most important thing. Relationships are reciprocal and the idea of 'give and take' still holds true for many. Community researchers can understand the nuances, the make-up of the community and they reveal rich insights into the lives of any community.

'Local knowledge'

Having the 'local knowledge' is an essential skill that researchers should look to develop in order to undertake ethnographic research. Reading about communities in academic books is one thing, but experiencing the community first-hand is a distinct advantage. The way I normally approach a new study site is to visit the study location, preferably taking a leisurely walk, walking through the streets, going into shops or just getting the feel of the place.

There are many alternatives; for example, in Bradford there are a number of Sunday markets taking place and they are a great way to find out what is going on in the neighbourhood. Hundreds of people attend (especially when Eid festival is fast approaching). Stalls sell everything from toiletries to loose cloth, from fruit and veg to fast food. It is a place of gathering and families come from many parts of Yorkshire to shop. By simply going along to a market, researchers can pick up much contextual information.

Melas

Another good way of 'mixing in' with the local community is to attend a mela. Many Asian areas around the UK hold annual melas which are attended by thousands of people (like the Sunday markets) and there can be literally hundreds of stalls. Live music, bouncy castles and face painting for children are popular activities. Melas take place during the summer and normally on a weekend. I always take business cards with me because there is always the possibility of making contact with individuals who may be able to help. Go along and enjoy! You can make plenty of contacts.

Eid festivals

Eid al-Fitr is a very busy time for Muslims. It is a collective religious celebration and events are held around the country to mark the end of the month of Fasting. Temporary market stalls are set up to cater for the needs of Muslims; it is a last-minute shopping spree for many and popular activities are mendhi (henna) painting and clothes shopping. It goes without saying food is an essential ingredient at the festivities. It is a time for Muslims to gather collectively, to 'hang out', enjoy street food and generally relax to mark the end of fasting.

Getting to know the locality is essential. I do quite a lot of preparatory work and initially I start by doing some background reading about the community. A good way of getting to know the community is to use public transport to get to a particular community centre. I remember doing fieldwork in one part of Leeds; I parked the car near the university and caught two buses to get to the centre. I had some time so I went into the local shop to buy a drink. A few exchanges of chit chat led to a conversation in which the shopkeeper remarked 'that I didn't look as if I lived around here'. I told him about the research study that I was working on and that I was here to conduct fieldwork. We chatted for nearly 30 minutes and in that time he talked about what it was like to live 'round here', problems faced by the local community and, in particular, the lack of employment prospects for young people and crime. Upon leaving, he wished me well and gave me some fruit for my lunch!

Similarly, on another occasion I remember arriving early for a pre-arranged interview and it was just around lunchtime. I popped into a local sandwich shop for my usual (tuna, sweetcorn sandwich!). The shopkeeper started a polite conversation, again as before, remarking that I looked as if I didn't live locally. I explained that I was working on a research study and was there to do a focus group interview at the local community centre. He started talking about the local community and some of the things that were happening here, the good and the bad. He started talking about himself, his family and the local Pakistani community.

It became a two-way conversation, discussing things that we had in common, for example the importance of family and the influence of the biraderi (kin). Much of the time I just listened to him as he served customers, benefiting from the knowledge that, had I taken the car instead of using public transport, I would have missed this one chance of striking up a conversation. I remember coming away with so much useful information about the community that I still remember it to this day.

At the beginning of fieldwork, information gathering is essential and, if you are an 'outsider', remember that understanding the local population is paramount, for example the main languages spoken, the dialects, the religious and cultural norms of the community. Talking to colleagues who are from the same community as the sample could be invaluable; they can talk to you about the neighbourhood, suitable places to approach and any individuals that could be helpful to the research study, more so the cultural etiquette. It is a natural outcome that, when 'outsiders' visit any community, members become almost 'suspicious', especially among close-knit communities like the Pakistanis, as their usual reactions are that the visitor may be an official from the government on an information-seeking mission. Assurance, especially when accompanied by a community researcher or a gatekeeper, can ease these fears.

Appearance is important, for example how one is dressed. A suit and tie may be inappropriate when visiting an inner city area that has a high crime rate, or when visiting a surestart or a community centre where one could inadvertently look like they are from the office of Works and Pensions. Matters can be made worse if they are seen entering a residential property, as prying neighbours often make their own mind up about a 'formally dressed individual entering the corner house'. This brings into question the issue of confidentiality. There should be few reasons to bring the visit into the public domain, and discretion is essential.

Another example is when visiting a community centre, where again one should be suitably dressed. On a warm, sunny day, for example, I would wear a pair of chinos and a white shirt (no tie!) so that one remains cool and aired, especially when one is going to be there for several hours. There are other 'rules' to be bear in mind, for example to make sure, as a male researcher, that you do not enter a room used by ladies unescorted. Sometimes you can be left alone to wander around the centre on your own, but just make sure you ask before you enter. A friendly, smiling and inviting style of approach is always the key; this also encourages service users and those working in the community centre to approach you and ask questions. Good social skills are learnt rather than taken for granted.

I have seen 'bad examples', including researchers who have come across as being unfriendly and closed. Of course, the natural reaction from the host centre has been likewise. Going with a colleague is always a good thing because you can bounce off ideas, and one of you can act as the observer and then 'unpick' your approach afterwards to (and, if negative) make sure you learn and improve next time.

Other bad examples include not forgetting to switch your mobile off upon entering the community centre! I recall one time when a colleague answered their mobile during a conversation and naturally this did not create a positive and professional image. Researchers have to remember that they are also representing the university in which they are employed. It should be a slick and professional engagement that leaves the service users (and community centre) wanting further engagement and be really interested in the research. Also, community centres have been around for many, many years and are visited by researchers all the time. To stand out from the rest is to be mindful of what is going on and one's manner. This seems like a lesson in social skills! But, after years of experience and talking to those in charge of community centres, what 'cuts the ice' is the individual rather than the commitment required from their centre.

What about the 'hard to reach'?

Reaching out to some groups in the community can be much more difficult to recruit from. Some are part of an invisible minority, whilst others are closely-knit groups that are difficult to reach out to. Gatekeepers are difficult to locate and get on board to help. Nevertheless, effort should be made to locate and offer the opportunity for individuals to participate in research in order to have a representative sample.

The following is a list (and not exhaustive by any means) of the 'hard to reach groups', e.g. individuals who are from an ethnic/Asian group (such as the Pakistani and Bangladeshis), females (from most ethnic backgrounds), young people and elderly (from all ethnic backgrounds). It also includes the 'minority within minority' groups who are often excluded from research studies due to the difficulty in recruiting participants, for example the Pushto-speaking females, individuals from LGB groups and those who have a disability. The list also includes participants who are engaged in home-based work (sewing, packing, etc.).

The difficulty around recruitment can be understanding the cultural and social barriers that stop researchers from accessing these groups, for example including cultural, religious and language reasons. Language is a good example; if the researchers did not adequately budget funds in the research grant for purposes of interpreting, then it becomes wholly difficult to access non-English groups. This is a communication failure.

The repeated message here is to do the preparatory homework to take these issues into account, otherwise individuals and groups can be overlooked. Funders perhaps should also have a responsibility to ensure that research is representative and adequate effort will be made by researchers to seek out groups that are largely overlooked because of difficulty around recruiting. However, it should not act as an excuse to marginalise perhaps the already marginalised.

Case study: A visit to a community centre

Over the years I have visited a number of community centres and voluntary organisations around Bradford for recruitment purposes. I can share some of my experiences here with researchers who may need to do the same at some point in their career.

'Selling the research'

The early career researcher will often find that they are left the task of recruiting from the community (or thrown in at the deep end!) often with little if, any help. If all other avenues have been explored and if the researcher is still having problems in recruiting a sufficient number of participants to a study, I suggest contacting managers at community centres. The important rule here is that this activity is about face to face communication. Sending e-mails and letters will often go answered and they come across as being impersonal; time is spent in preparing the text and then simply either printed out or copied into an e-mail and sent to numerous potential host organisations. It is an activity that requires the least amount of resources. The reasons for this are understandable given that most community centres have only a small number of paid workers, often relying on volunteers to keep the centre running. Time and resources are often stretched and little time is left to reply to a blanket e-mail or letter.

What is needed in abundance is 'initiative and flare' to do things differently, to think independently and also the flexibility to be able to think differently by the senior research team. It depends upon the senior research team members and, if they do not allow this, then the fieldworker will revert to what *is* being allowed. Generally, the longer the senior researchers spend being a fieldworker, the more acceptable and open they are to suggestions, especially from those who are more experienced in fieldwork.

So, once the researcher gets the go-ahead, I strongly suggest a visit to the community centre in person. Upon arrival, ask to see the manager or the person in charge, introduce yourself and explain the reason for the visit; then, if time allows, speak to the person in charge, preferably in a quiet room (because what you want is their undivided attention and not to be disturbed). Or, if he/she does not have available time, make a follow-up appointment to return. Remember to take your business card, leaflets and any other written information about the study so that you can leave these with the person to read at their leisure. Never forget to leave contact details with the person in charge. I have seen this happen on a number occasions. For those who are on a part-time contract and those who are away from their office, they should be prepared to leave their mobile number in case they need to be contacted. Leaving a message on the office answering message means it could be days or perhaps even weeks before you hear the message, and it could be an opportunity lost.

When visiting, I strongly suggest that you have a folder with all the essential information about the study; it shows good preparation and also you will not be rushing around 'digging' out various bits of information from your bag! Making a visit to the community centre requires a lot of planning and foresight. Essentially, they want to put a face to the research (letters and emails do not do this) and you, as a researcher, should be looking for rapport and trust because, if they 'trust' you, they will trust the research.

Personal experience shows that clarity is essential given that the researcher probably has about five minutes (at most) to create a good impression. After the introductions, the person in charge will either entertain you further or simply say 'no', e.g. their service users would not be interested in the research study. It comes as a surprise when I tell my colleagues that research is about 'selling' the project to participants and organisations. Creating a positive vibe is essential; if they see the researcher enthused in the research, this will go a long way in creating the right environment and interaction. Good body language is also an essential ingredient, and dress code has been discussed elsewhere in the book. These are things that need to be borne in mind.

Always remember that you as a researcher are an 'invited guest' in the community centre and that you are asking them to help you in your endeavour. Irrespective of how 'desperate' you are of needing to recruit participants in the research study, it's essential you do not come across as being 'needy'. Always allow space and time to the recipient to decide whether they can help you or not as it's difficult for anyone to make an on the spot decision. Perhaps they need to discuss with the board or individuals, or they need to ask their service users whether they would be interested in taking part in the research. Also, they would most probably want to discuss the proposed research with their governing body.

If you get the 'go ahead' from the community centre, one needs to be well-planned; the researcher needs to take the time to explain the research, the purpose and the benefits. The researcher needs to be clear whether time or resource commitments are needed from the host organisation and this certainly would be a question that will be asked by the host organisation. Also, they will probably ask questions on payment and whether they (or the service users who take part) will receive any payment in return for their time. As researchers will be well aware, payments are never made to prospective participants, as simply providing lunch and refreshments to those taking part is sufficient. A point to bear in mind is, if you have agreed to provide lunch, then you should make sure food is appropriate for the clientele. I always ask the host organisation or service users what they would prefer; generally, however, it is good to remember that, for example, elderly Pakistani people tend to prefer traditional and 'warm' foods such as pakoras, samosas, rice and roti rather than cold sandwiches, while other groups may also prefer these foods in addition to cold sandwiches or a meat variety.

It can take time (and patience) to develop a good working relationship with community organisations. Personal experience shows that managers at community centres are good at remembering individuals and this is great if you need to go back to them at some future date. A point to remember is that most staff at community centres are busy, often volunteers, so if you give them some time to accommodate you then you will be off to a good start!

'You only get one bite at the cherry'

The task of recruiting individuals to studies can be 'tricky'; if one approaches this with a planned strategy and thought, then it should be a relatively 'smooth' experience. You will come across as being confident and in charge of the situation. Nothing is more valuable than experience and this becomes clearly evident as time progresses. Each situation is different and requires an approach that is both adaptable and accommodating.

A point worth bearing in mind is that it would be naïve for the researcher to think that they can simply turn up at the community centre and quickly be introduced to 'loads' of research participants who would be eager to participate. Secondly, 'rejection' should not be taken personally; for all sorts of reasons, the person in charge on the day of your visit may feel it is inappropriate for the researcher to recruit from his/her service users. They may be in the middle of re-organisation, training or cuts in their funding. Certain times of the year are always a busy period for community centres; April is usually a month when funding is allocated, while Christmas is also a busy period as a number of personnel will be celebrating the festive period, or simply taking time off to spend with their children or loved ones.

The month of fasting usually means that the majority of Muslim workers at the community centres will be either away on holiday or on a reduced number of hours for the duration of the fasting month, thus less likely to commit. This has a 'knock on' effect on recruitment, for example during these times there may be fewer service users in attendance preparing for the festivities. Especially if one needs to recruit older people, the winter months may mean that they stay away at home. If one bears such issues in mind, then one should delay recruiting over certain time periods.

The worst scenario (and one that happens to all researchers at some point!) is that you get a rejection; it would then be a good opportunity to re-examine the approach and technique. Could he/she have done anything differently? For example, perhaps the language they used with the person in charge of the centre was too technical? Perhaps it was in the way they explained the study? I do not, however, prepare a script – perhaps a number of points (in bullet form) that I want to get across in a couple of minutes. It depends upon the situation; some may enjoy all the 'ins and outs' of the research from an explanation about ethics committees to R&D, whereas, for others, it may be too much, especially if they are in-patients.

Adapting your approach according to the needs of your clientele are essential prerequisites. Overall, irrespective of clientele, one should try to keep it simple. I think plain simple English 'always rules' and is always the best policy. Some researchers never seem to adapt or understand human nature and talk as if they are reading from a prepared script, whether they are talking to a renowned professor or lay person on the street. All said, there will be times when a certain amount of technical language will be used, for example studies involving clinical trials. As they say, practice makes perfect; one should go through the essential points, replacing the more difficult, complicated words with simpler language if possible.

This should all be considered when writing information sheets, consent forms and study material. Team meetings should involve going through such material and seeing whether any points can be made simpler. The purpose of the information sheet is to explain the study rather than a long technical essay which, in reality, few will read properly before consenting to take part. It is important for researchers to understand how this will work in practice and in the real world.

An appropriate scenario is that the prospective participant will listen to a verbal explanation about the study, followed by the researcher going through the information sheet, and then having to listen to the researcher going through the consent form, and all of this even before they start completing a lengthy study questionnaire. That's a lot of information for anyone to take! This could take upwards of thirty minutes from start to finish. This may well lead to the prospective participant saying 'no' upon realising the time commitment involved, especially if they are in a hospital situation, perhaps waiting for surgery, or had a medical procedure some days earlier and are not feeling fully fit.

Avoiding some obvious pitfalls

Preparation is the key. If it is the first time you are visiting a community centre and if you are in a position to take a colleague who is knowledgeable with you for support, then do so. You're perhaps likely to forget to mention something about the research, whereas your friend or colleague could help out here. Another good technique is to prepare a short 'script' (couple of bullet points) and to make sure all the essentials of the research are included, for example the inclusion criteria (this could be service users who speak a specific language or a dialect, from a particular part of Bradford or Pakistan, or users who are suffering from a particular condition say diabetes) and the exclusion criteria (those who are under 16). The important thing to remember here is that those working in community centres or those in charge may not know about research, so one has to prepare a layperson's version (given they probably do not have the time for the researcher to talk through a long spiel). It would be a good idea to take along (if you have them) information sheets, consent forms, or a discussion guide in case they may want to have a read and ask questions. The important thing to remember is that, essentially, it will be the job of the researcher to ensure sufficient information is passed.

The approach: face to face or telephone?

I often get asked the question (both from the experienced and those who are new to research) the best way to approach community centres (gatekeepers and community leaders). In my experience, the majority of researchers will draft a letter (it is nearly always addressed as 'Dear Sir/Madam' rather than the person's name), outlining the nature of the study, 'type' of respondents required, as well as the inclusion and the exclusion criteria; they will enclose the information sheet and then send it to the community centre. There will be a pre-printed label on the envelope. If the researcher does not receive a reply, they will wait for two weeks before sending another reminder. All of this is impersonal. In the vast majority of cases, they will never receive a reply! As mentioned earlier, community centres often only have a few paid workers and rely on volunteers to run the centre on a day-to-day basis. There are also often financial pressures.

Researchers also overlook the fact that community centres receive letters from researchers and other parties requesting some form of action on a weekly basis and usually they don't have the time to reply. Personally, I very much favour the personal visit to the community centre as opposed to sending letters through post. It has a distinct advantage: since research is about 'people'; the person in charge can talk to the researcher face to face and go through the practicalities and the sample size, etc. All of this is much easier done face to face rather than on the phone (or worse, through the post). Also, people are less likely to say 'no' when they have sat talking to you for any length of time. Face to face communication allows the researcher to develop a bond and to relate to the host centre; however, for some (even experienced) researchers, this is something they will probably never entertain.

In my experience, the best time to visit a community centre is about an hour or so after they open; for example, if the centre opens at 9am, the researcher should try to get there by about 10 or 10.30am. I say this because the main disadvantage to arriving too early is that they will probably be getting things ready for the day, for example setting up sports equipment. However, most probably the centre manager will be catching up with colleagues about the daily rota. Thus, by arriving a little later means you will miss the early hustle and bustle and have an excellent chance of speaking to the manager.

The researcher, upon arrival at the community centre, should report to the reception desk (however, one should bear in mind that some centres may not have a reception, so the best thing here is to speak to someone who works there). If you ascertain that the manager has not arrived or will be unavailable for day, the best thing to do is to leave your contact card and ask when he/she will be in, thus making a follow-up appointment.

If you do state a date/time for your return, then one should always keep to it since most likely they will be expecting you. People are always likely to respond better when you come across as being approachable and pleasant.

Some colleagues think that, if they are unable to speak to a person in charge at the initial visit, they will be disappointed, e.g. they are unable to speak to the centre manager/person in charge. However, I view this as an advantage because, if you have arranged an appointment with the reception desk, it means that a) you will speak to someone in charge and in authority, thus a person who is able to make a decision; b) you will have the person's undivided attention, say, for thirty minutes at the follow-up meeting and, hopefully, will not be interrupted; and c) it should mean that you will be more relaxed and comfortable when you talk about the proposed research study. I can say with confidence that, of all the places I have visited for purposes of data collection, I have always been given the opportunity to discuss the research either in the office of the manager or somewhere quiet (sometimes this was in the gym room, other times on the balcony!).

Although there is no hard and fast rule, what I have found is that the most successful researchers (and fieldworkers) should be flexible and adaptable in their approach. As mentioned elsewhere, imagination, flair and a good open personality means you will stand apart from all those gone before you and thus create a good chance of recruiting from the host organisation.

Knowing the service users

On a personal level, I always enjoy visiting community centres, voluntary organisations, etc. Perhaps I am naturally inquisitive and interested in how individuals are part of a larger community (particularly 'Asian' communities).

The important thing to bear in mind about community centres is that each one is 'different' and, although their doors are always open, we find that they usually cater for the needs of a particular group. For example, in Bradford there are numerous centres and voluntary organisations catering for Pakistani, Indian, Bangladeshi, white/English, elderly and disabled groups. The message here is do your homework! Understand the local population and hopefully you will have some valuable insight into the service users. Common mistakes that researchers make here are not realising the age group of service users, the languages spoken or the ethnic/cultural makeup of service users.

Community centres are an important information resource for people. For some, they are a 'lifeline' offering services such as advice on social security benefits, help with filling in forms, helping the unemployed to look for work, offering advice on money and debt to name just a few. They offer so much more to service users, for example teaching English to non-English speakers.

There is a whole host of other classes being run throughout the year including sewing, self-defence and computer classes. Since community centres are based in the local neighbourhood, they offer individuals (particularly females) the chance to enrol and make a real difference to their lives; also, they do not have to travel any distance to learn. The UK has been accommodating all cultures and religions by helping and encouraging individuals (and communities) to become part of this great nation, particularly for individuals to learn English, which is a prerequisite for 'fitting in' and to simply interact with the indigenous population. There is perhaps no country in the world that spends a substantial amount of money-holding classes in English and in neighbourhoods for the benefit of individuals and all of this is evident in the community centres.

I always enjoying visiting community centres so, even though I and my parents were from Pakistan, I am always interested to hear about the 'Pakistani' culture, which is not homogenous (for further discussion see Din, 2006), especially when I visit a centre where the majority of service users are Pakistanis. They often talk about childhood memories about what it was like growing up in Pakistan (e.g. the building of the Mangla Dam and the subsequent migration to New Mirpur, biraderi), the importance of maintaining 'izzat', or honour (for further in-depth discussion see Din, 2006). Also, their early married life, when they first came to the UK, and also the hopes and dreams they had not only for their immediate family members but for the whole Pakistani community, in addition to making a positive contribution to the host society; the pressures of being 'successful', to studying hard and gaining good employment. For some families, many have seen the fruits of their hard labour, while for other parents they have become disappointed and disillusioned, mostly with their own community.

Much of this is narrative, which I enjoy listening and responding to with my own experiences of being a first generation Pakistani growing up in Bradford. Having experienced the early settlement of Pakistanis in Bradford and how culture (and religion) played a significant role in defining family and community life, it becomes a two-way conversation.

The atmosphere in the centre is nearly always relaxed and welcoming. The great thing about the centres is that most will allow you to talk to their users freely. I often sit with service users over a cup of tea or lunch talking about wherever the conversation leads. For example, one community centre I frequently visit is based on the outskirts of Bradford and, if I am recruiting there late morning, I always get invited to their luncheon (and I never say 'no'!). Another is based in the inner city; they serve tea and coffee in the morning and, again, I get invited to sit and enjoy a drink and the company.

I think it's a great way to break down barriers. For most service users, they would never have come across a researcher and would be naturally inquisitive both about what a 'researcher' does as well as being interested in 'you' as a person. When I go along to any community centre (or a place of gathering), I nearly always get asked about my family, my parents, about family in Pakistan – in fact, a whole host of questions. This can come across as being impersonal to the 'outsider', but to the Pakistani community, particularly among the elderly Pakistani, they like to know about 'you' as a person before they are ready to be responsive and help you in your research. Research is about being personal, to share information and to ask questions freely.

Recruiting individuals to research studies

Hopefully you have got the 'go-ahead' from the community centre to approach their service users, so what's next? Well, now the work really begins! The (difficult) task of recruiting individuals to the study starts. I think it's appropriate to use a case study of one community centre I frequently visit for purposes of recruitment. This particular community centre is based on the outskirts of Bradford, serving primarily Pakistani service users. Without doubt, this community centre is a 'focal point' for the locals and this is easy to see having visited many times. There are a number of activities taking place during the day and in the evening. They hold English classes for females (and males) who have arrived from

Pakistan and speak little or no English. In the evening, young people (both boys and girls) go along to the centre and have the opportunity to engage in sports activities such as table tennis and badminton (they are free to participate in), as well as having the opportunity to 'chill out' with friends in a safe environment. Refreshments can also be bought at reduced prices. It serves primarily the local Pakistani community. The centre is located in a 'deprived' area with a high rate of unemployment, especially youth unemployment. It is also a high crime rate area, with fewer children leaving school with 5 GCSEs and less likely to go on to university.

The centre is particularly important for its elderly users as it provides a transport service in order for them to get to the sessions. For most elderly service users, it is the only time they are able to venture out of their home since most have mobility restrictions and a number of them suffer from long-term conditions such as diabetes and heart conditions. Users have access to a small gym, or they can watch a movie and play board games. However, most just use it for the purposes of socialising and meeting friends they have made.

It is a good idea to visit the centre and a have a good look around before approaching potential participants. This has the distinct advantage of allowing the researcher to 'get to know' the place. Even at this stage, there is nothing to be lost in approaching service users who may be curious when they see a face they have not seen before (never miss an opportunity!).

If you do not have the time or the opportunity to do the above, then the way I approach the task of recruiting participants is to go along to all the sessions being held at the centre and talk to as many service users as possible. However, you don't want to give the impression you are lost! Be prepared to ask for a guided tour as this allows the guide to introduce you to the person in charge of the class and/or potential participants as you go from one location to another.

There is no 'hard and fast' shortcut and it takes a lot of time, effort and confidence on the part of the researcher to talk to individuals. A face to face interview allows you to explain the research and answer any questions the interviewee may have. On occasions, when I have run out of time, I simply go along to the next session and pick up where I left off. It is important to make a note of who you have spoken to and whether they would be interested in taking part. I repeat this until everyone has had the opportunity to participate – and, I iterate, 'everyone'. Research is about giving as many people the opportunity to participate as possible, as the 'opportunities' are in abundance for the committed researcher conducting fieldwork.

You may run out of time or some participants may prefer to be interviewed at another location. I have been invited to conduct the interview at the home of participants on numerous occasions. Be prepared for this to happen. Following on from your chat at the centre, arrange a suitable date and time. The best approach is to be as flexible as possible. In order to do this, you should have remembered to take your work diary, bearing in mind that you may have to cancel other pre-arranged meetings at work (you should have alerted your manager that this may happen before leaving the office).

Timing is crucial, and the important consideration is not to get interrupted during the interview. A good time to arrange the interview is after the staff have done their early morning chores, for example cooking and cleaning, while others may have children and need to drop them off to school, so bear this in mind. I generally find that arranging a morning interview at, say, 10.30am works well; this gives you about an hour and a half to conduct the interview before they need to collect their children from school or carry out other chores. Since the interview takes place at the home of the participant, it is an environment that is comfortable for them; the surroundings ensure that they will be relaxed – an important ingredient for a successful interview.

Location of interview: place of one's work

The aim is to get the participant(s) to relax and feel at ease (although you may be feeling uneasy!). It is worth remembering that, even if you are an experienced researcher, most participants would not have been interviewed before so you need to be prepared. On the day of the interview it is best to arrive before the participant to ensure the setting is as comfortable as it can be, for example to make sure the seating is pleasant, the lighting is good, perhaps open a window if it is a nice sunny day! Another good idea is to have some cold drinks on the side table. It is about breaking down the formality of the interview and so much about creating a dialogue rather than the process being prescriptive. Over time, one can build up a list of things one should do at the pre-interview stage and, above else, those things that work. If done well, it shows ingenuity, learnt skills and professionalism on the part of the researcher.

'Ethics' of the interview (Din, 2006)

Anonymity is difficult to ensure when participants may know each other. Those taking part may live on the same street or they could be related. The location of the focus group also needs to be carefully planned. Also, issues such as location of the interview are important, for example holding a focus group in the local community centre can be unsuitable. 'Asian' community centres tend to be used mainly by men, and Pakistani women are often reluctant to attend unfamiliar or male-orientated surroundings.

There are other issues that need to be taken into account. The date and time of the interview is important. For example, researchers must avoid making contact with Pakistani participants at Namaz time (there are five Namaz a day at various times), Thursday evenings when special prayers are said and during Jumma (Friday prayers held during early afternoon). While other special occasions take place once a year, one also needs to be aware of Ramadan (Fasting) and Eid. This is particularly busy time for Pakistanis and researchers should avoid making contact during this time – or, even better, avoid any contact with this sample group. A letter instead could be sent explaining that the research team wishes to conduct an interview with a member of the household, but feel that it is inappropriate to arrange this during Ramadan and will make contact after Eid. If the initial contact is made face-to-face and time for Namaz happens to overlap with the interview (something that may be unavoidable), then it is expected that the researcher who is part of this community should join in the Namaz. A researcher who is not part of the community should be aware of the time of the Namaz and allow time accordingly.

It is important to be prepared and adapt as circumstances change. Something that can be overlooked by researchers is the fact that not all Pakistanis (or, indeed, all Asians) are the same and/or will have the same practices.

It is essential to understand 'Pakistani etiquette'. If the researcher conducting the interview is from outside the community, then it advisable for him/her to talk to one of his/her Pakistani colleagues to ask questions and explain the 'dos and don'ts'. The interview starts when the first contact is made. When entering the participant's house, it is polite to offer to remove one's shoes and exchange salaam (greetings) with the participant. In the case of a male researcher, a firm handshake with the male participant is normal. If there are males present, the researcher must shake hands and exchange salaam in order of importance, starting with the eldest first. If there are females present, then the male researcher must exchange salaam first with the lady(s) and then, by shaking hands, starting with the eldest male. In the case of a female researcher, she must salaam the lady(s) first, normally a handshake and/or hug, followed by salaam with any males present. It is customary to sit down without being asked by the participant, since the guest should treat the 'home like his home'. This is followed by further customary salaams and asking about one's health and about any children the participant may have (if the researcher is aware of this). Other common topics of discussion are Pakistan and current affairs.

Where the interview is not gender-matched (for example, male researcher and female interviewee), then under no circumstances should the researcher ask questions about the participant's female siblings. In this case, the male researcher should only speak when he is spoken to. This is made easier when a female researcher interviews a male participant. She is often treated as a 'daughter' and most issues can be discussed such as siblings. As part of this trust-building process, the researcher must be able to talk about what is regarded as being 'personal information' in the Western sense, e.g. talking about one's marital status, siblings, background of the spouse and parents. It is customary to be open and genuine in a community where little is kept hidden. In this situation, both the participant and the researcher are being interviewed by each other.

Building rapport between the researcher and the participant is essential. To make them feel at ease and relaxed, and to encourage a natural discussion between two individuals, cultural sensitivity is paramount. Rapport means that the researcher is often asked questions about his family, including his/her age, whether or not he/she is married and, if applicable, if he/she has any children, names of his/her parents and grandparents, where they come from in Pakistan, names of uncles and aunts and what they do.

Hospitality is an integral part of the Pakistani community, thus taking tea and even dinner should be accepted when offered. Hospitality should not be refused since it is likely to cause offence. If the researcher is younger than the participant, then he/she should serve tea, again starting with the eldest male/female first. This is all part of the introduction stage.

Most people have some experience of being interviewed, often in a job interview situation, but fewer people are interviewed for research purposes. For most, it is a totally new and alien situation. Often, the research participant is unsure in terms of how to answer questions. Others might 'guess' the correct answer by saying what the researcher wants to hear. This is similar to being in a classroom situation where the child is second-guessing what the teacher wants to hear. Answering questions, often in a structured way, is difficult for most and the researcher needs to explain and discuss this with the participant.

The researcher should also ask the participant in what form he/she requires further correspondence to be made, for example by letter, telephone, or email (depending on the literacy levels of the individual), while others may prefer to receive communication to be made through a third party. It is also important to know which dialect the participant speaks and to provide correspondence in that language or dialect.

Any communication between the researcher and the participant should be in English, Urdu or in any other dialect (letters, etc.) and/or recorded on audio tape in case the participant is unable to read. It is important to be aware of language issues and the many dialects spoken. For example, most Pakistanis speak Azad Kashmiri Punjabi. The golden rule is that each participant will be different and the researcher needs to do 'research on the participant'.

Researchers need to be aware of other issues, for example how the sample group would be contacted raises further issues, confidentiality being one of these. If contact is made by telephone, one needs to know what would happen if the 'elder' answers, which is what normally happens amongst the Pakistanis. The 'elder' can be the father, mother, brother, the husband or the in-laws. He/she must be convinced of the purpose of the research and would normally request to read the topic guide and/or even meet the researcher. It is this person who will often grant access to their family members as he/she is the spokesperson for the family. The question is, who is consenting to take part, the elder or the person concerned? Participants such as unmarried girls and spouses from Pakistan are particularly difficult to recruit. Taking into account the above concerns, for most it is impolite to simply telephone and introduce the research. Whenever possible, the initial contact should be made face-to-face, where potential participants can put a face to the name and the purpose of the research can be explained.

The place of the interview is crucial. If the interview is arranged to take place in the home of the participant, then researchers need to be aware that family members could come into the room. What if they decide to stay and contribute? It is not acceptable to ask family members to leave the room or, indeed, ask to be left alone while the interview is being conducted. This would go against the cultural norms of the Pakistani community where secrecy is frowned upon.

The researcher is a guest and should conduct the interview at a place where the participant will feel comfortable and at ease. These circumstances can be awkward for the participant, where he/she may feel cajoled or obliged into continuing the interview (not by the researcher) but by the 'third party' present. In this case, the researcher should allow – even encourage – the interview to be rearranged to take away the responsibility from the participant, particularly when the spouse is present.

It is normally made clear at the outset that the interview will be conducted in private to ensure confidentiality, but the reality is often different. Researchers need to be careful when asking for consent from the participant in the presence of third parties. It is common for an 'unwanted guest' such as a relative to be visiting, or a family member to be present at the time of the interview.

The question is whether the interview should take place. The 'unwanted guest' could contribute to the interview and to whatever is being discussed. The focus of the interview can often change depending on the contribution made by the 'unwanted guest'. But how valid is the data collected in these circumstances? Is it ethical and is it confidential? Some would say the interview should be rearranged for another time. However, to do so we would be overlooking the norms of the community in question. The situation is culturally specific. We think the 'unwanted guest' can be excused from the interview room, but this would be from a Western perspective whereas, in this community, whoever is present at the time can remain present and is allowed to contribute. It is not considered polite to ask the 'guest' to leave and should not be suggested to the participant; after all, the researcher is also a guest in the participant's house. The 'interview' is often along the lines of a communal discussion as opposed to being one-to-one. Western research methods are sometimes not applicable when conducting research on the Pakistani community.

Leaving the house after the interview can raise other issues such as prying neighbours and relatives who often reside nearby, as is the case of the Pakistanis. The intrusive neighbour, who enquires about the researcher, can lead to divulging the nature of the interview unwillingly and, in some cases, the participant should not be interviewed. As pointed out earlier, the location of the interview should be left to the discretion of the participant.

'Language' of the interview

If the researcher speaks a community language then, at some point during their research career, they will be expected to conduct an interview or focus group in a community ('home') language. To do this properly takes a lot of preparation and practice and, above all else, to make sure they have the necessary skills to do this effectively. For example, for those who speak Urdu this could be a relatively easy process; Urdu is the national language of Pakistan, and the national newspaper and governmental documentation are written in Urdu. Discussions, guides and study materials can be translated with little problem. However, if the participant speaks a 'dialect', then this becomes a much more difficult task.

As a case example, most of the Pakistanis living in the UK originate from Mirpur, a region in Azad Kashmir (Pakistan) and speak a dialect called 'Mirpuri' (others may call this Kashmiri or Punjabi; there are many other common dialects spoken in Pakistan including Hindko, Pushto and Pothwari). Most words do not have an equivalent in Mirpuri, thus translation becomes a problem. The Mirpuri dialect essentially consists of words borrowed from Urdu, and English words such as 'door', 'window', 'car', or 'pen' are frequently used in place of Mirpuri words.

For the bilingual researcher, this creates all sorts of problems wherein you can have a written discussion guide in English and Urdu, but one cannot have a written version in Mirpuri. In reality, the bilingual researcher will 'translate' questions as they go along. The advice for the bilingual researcher is that they should do a quick 'mapping exercise' and ask the gatekeeper or the community centre manager the dialects spoken by service users. However, bear in mind that sometimes further clarity may be required; if this happens, then I would approach some of the service users and simply hold a conversation in the dialect.

'Barriers': Gender issues and the community

One of the questions I get asked is how does a male researcher access and recruit female respondents from a community setting? Again, taking a case example of the Pakistani community, although the short answer is that it can be very difficult to access female groups if you are a male researcher, good planning can help make this difficult task less arduous. Knowing the community in which the sample will derive is essential and different groups (within the 'Pakistani community' there are many regional groups, for example Pushto speakers) will require a different approach.

The best approach (and one that always works for me) is that I will visit one of the community centres (other places I may visit are places of worship or elderly day centres) and try and get a female gatekeeper on board to help identify potential participants to the study. This should make approaching respondents easier because the initial introductions are done by the gatekeeper (while you as the researcher need only introduce yourself at this point!). So, whilst being escorted by the gatekeeper, I normally keep a log in my mind of the service users who come across as being receptive to the study. Following on from this, the next stage would be to go round and talk to individuals.

As an example, one of the more difficult groups to 'reach' and recruit to studies are young Pakistani females, particularly Pushto speakers who originate from the north-west frontier of Pakistan. Access to this group is difficult because they are traditionally a closed group, particularly to outsiders (and males). Although in the past I have recruited from this group, I have done so by using female gatekeepers from the community to help with access issues (otherwise it would have been impossible).

Going back a step (and only recommended to the most determined of researchers!), there is a lot of ‘ground work’ to do. I start by having at least one in-depth preliminary meeting with the gatekeeper to explain the ‘ins and outs’ of research and answer any questions that they may have. Through experience, you ‘get a feel’ and understand whether service users would be happy to talk to a male researcher. If resources allow, there may be an opportunity to employ a female community researcher to help with tasks (however, from experience most research studies would not have included the cost in the original grant funding for the use of employing a community researcher). If this is the case, then recruiting Pakistani (Asian) female participants may become a problem, but one can only try and it’s worth giving it a go, since often their experiences are overlooked by the community as well as research studies because of the reasons given.

Summary

This research sets out some of the essentials of doing research on a minority ethnic community and, in this case, the Pakistanis. By reading this chapter, it is envisaged it will help researchers to be aware of the issues that may arise during recruitment and ways in which they may be tackled. Much of the advice and suggestions given have been tried and trusted by the author, but invariably each researcher will have to find their own solutions to ‘hurdles’ and ‘barriers’ they will undoubtedly come across during their research carriers.

Essentially, research should be seen as giving a ‘voice’ to research participants (and the community they may be part of). Through ethnographic research, we not only learn about individuals but also their community. At the end, you should get a general consensus as to commonality coming out of the research, a rich tapestry of inter-linked and interrelated experiences that give a powerful voice to the participants.

Researchers are in a privileged position because they often hear about life stories that are contextual to the research. I feel privileged when this happens because this can be considered as breaking down barriers between the researcher and participant; sometimes this happens, whilst at other times it can be a struggle to get any form of dialogue going. Hopefully, things discussed in this chapter should make this a rare occurrence.

There are many 'essential' skills needed to be a successful community researcher. For example, having the skills to listen in a non-judgemental manner is essential. At the same time, it is about listening to their narrative; at times, this can be relevant to the research study and, at other times, it can be about their home life, about their community or some difficulty they are going through.

It is also important to bear in mind that it might be the first time they have been interviewed. Some researchers prefer to ask questions in a structured way; however, I prefer the method that allows participants the flexibility in their response (but this depends upon the research and the methodology to be used). Starting off with 'easy' introductory questions is a good way to get the participant thinking about the research study and, hopefully, 'open up' to more inquisitive questions later. Over the years, I have found that much of the open dialogue happens after the 'formal' interview and it's the stage where most participants feel relaxed.

The key personal specifications of a researcher I would say are as follows: friendly, open and someone who is genuinely interested in the individual (and the community) as opposed to someone who is there just to collect the data for the purposes of publishing papers and career development. Potential participants and gatekeepers can sense this very quickly and are more likely to say 'no'. For them, the concern is that the researcher should be genuinely interested in the community.

Conducting family interviews

Interviewing participants at home can be very different from conducting interviews in a community setting. Over the years I have conducted numerous interviews in the home of the participant and, although all interviews are different, conducting interviews in the 'home setting' can need extra planning and foresight. To illustrate this, I will use a case scenario to illustrate some of the practical difficulties and helpful pointers to aid the researcher if they conduct an interview at home.

About 10 years ago, I was conducting fieldwork in an inner city area of a Yorkshire town. Previously, I had visited a community centre to recruit older Pakistanis to a study looking at the importance of communication between patients and healthcare professionals. I recruited a participant who was in her 60s and who was happy to take part (always a relief for the field researcher when you get the golden 'yes' from a participant). As I was preparing to go through the information sheet, I was informed by the supervisor of the community centre that they would be closing for the day. Naturally disappointed, but not wanting to lose the participant (the look on my face said it all, I think), the lady suggested that, if it was acceptable to me, I could conduct the interview in her home. I naturally jumped at the invitation!

The interview was arranged for the following week. I arrived on time and the door was answered by the lady's daughter-in-law. After the introduction, I went inside (always be prepared to remove one's shoes in the hallway – as an indicator, you will normally see outside shoes in the hallway). I was then taken to a rather large lounge room, which had members of the lady's family present (I wasn't really surprised to find family members present). In the room, the lady's husband, two sons and the daughter-in-law were watching television. I was greeted by the male members of the family with a handshake (always shake hands with male members of the family, generally the eldest first, so in this situation the husband of the participant followed by the participant's two sons). Like in all cultures, it shows sincerity and friendship and the breaking down of barriers.

The general chit-chat with the family members was followed by an explanation of the research study; all the family members remained in the room, whilst I went through the information sheet and consent forms. I did explain that the interview was a 'one-to-one'; however, the participant felt that it was good to have family members in the room whilst I conducted the interview. From experience this has happened on a number of occasions, where the one-to-one interview becomes a 'family interview'. It is difficult to ask family members to leave the room. Again, preparation is the key: this scenario should be raised during the team meetings to decide what would be the best possible solution. In my case, the participant answered the questions, but with contributions from family members, particularly on questions around interpreting and translating (the participant did not speak English). Personally, I found the contribution made by family members interesting and informative, building a much broader picture of the participant; for example, how the participant is supported by members of her family in various settings, including help with translation when attending an appointment at the hospital, home help doing everyday things like preparing a meal and help with washing.

Similarly, in Pakistan researchers will find that interviews conducted at the home of the participant will have members of the biraderi in attendance; they are often curious, but one will find that they will be more than happy to engage in the conversation. Experience is the key; the researcher needs to play it by ear (personally, I 'go with the flow'), adapting to the situation in order to get the best out of the interview.

The interview has to be 'user-friendly' and adaptable (remembering that the researcher is the guest of the participant). The general rules are to keep the interaction open, friendly and fluid by allowing the participant to dictate who is allowed to sit during the interview and their level of involvement. For the new researcher, much of this may sound like a daunting task, but it is worth remembering that this is meant to be a learning experience; the more you do, the better prepared you will become. I enjoy doing 'family interviews' as everyone in the room has a viewpoint or experience that they would like to share, and everyone is given an opportunity to contribute (usually the elder gets the first opportunity to contribute).

Benefits of research studies

One of the most 'tricky' questions that a researcher is asked (certainly in my experience) is how the research will benefit service users in the community centre, or what will they gain from participating. There isn't an easy answer; for example, if the research is examining the language needs of Pakistani diabetic patients in Bradford, then those who provide resources such as interpreters would be better placed to understand the language needs of this community and therefore resources could be better targeted.

Further, experience suggests that participants are wanting to hear 'benefits'. What is the big outcome? How will all of this change their situation or experience? If they are hospital patients they will naturally be thinking about whether their participation will lead to an improved service, or even perhaps more staff being made available. There has to be a positive outcome for participants, one which is realistic and obtainable. Ivory tower research fails to convince anyone. We rarely ask participants and communities what they think of research. Questions that perhaps need to be answered are: Do participants think research studies serve a purpose? Are some types of research more beneficial than others? Or is it all just an academic exercise?

The following is a section of my previous research (Din, 2008) wherein I asked participants about their attitudes and the value of research.

Participating in research: viewpoint from Bradford

My earlier research (Din, 2008) respondents mentioned the importance of having available 'time' in order to participate in research. That researchers need to allow respondents sufficient time to participate in research is of generic importance and this issue is discussed in depth earlier. For example, the importance of (as in the present study) not contacting respondents during prayer times, during the month of Ramadan or during the Eid festivals is important,

> "Yes, if I have the time" (female, aged 49)

This is understandable, since respondents were either working outside of the home or working from home, for example sewing clothes or packing cards, which was labour-intensive. This was in addition to running the household and doing everyday chores such as cooking or shopping. As explained in my previous research (Cullingford and Din, 2006; Din 2006), researchers need to be aware that, like all populations, certain times can be inappropriate to contact respondents, particularly when making contact with Pakistanis given that most older Pakistanis read Namaz five times a day and, during the month of Ramadan, most would be unavailable (Din, 2008).

Those who had the knowledge to access health information (because of language, etc.) were thought of as being educated. Information was seen as a tool and a mechanism for holding 'power'. One way to obtain this was through research, as pointed out by a number of respondents in this study, through developing contacts (family and friends), through the media and through more formal networks such as health professionals (as we will see later),

> "Information is power. People should help, if they can more people would help with health research if they had the time" (female, aged 56)

A feature of that research was asking participants to talk about the research process both before and after the interview. This is rarely done by researchers. Most respondents (16/18 of the Bradford sample and 8/10 of the Mirpur sample) had not been interviewed before for research purposes. The following were typical of responses received from the Bradford interviewees,

> "No one has ever interviewed me before" (female, aged 57)

> "I have not been interviewed before. I am happy to participate in doing research" (male, aged 59)

A small number of respondents have had some contact with researchers, for example at the local health centre,

> "Not really, when I am at the local centre I guess when ladies talk to me they look for gossip, is that research? I have answered questions at the doctor's surgery regarding my fitness levels by the Health Visitor" (female, aged 68)

Encouraging individuals to participate in research is paramount in order to understand attitudes and beliefs, particularly of those who are part of minority communities. Research allows individuals to learn about their own conditions as well as informing others about the pitfalls, for example about thinking about what they eat,

> "I like to help people, this research might help uncover the reasons why people eat the food they do and help people improve their diet and lifestyle" (male, aged 72)

Similarly, another said,

> "If I can help with the research you are doing I am happy to do so if this study can identify where Pakistani people's eating and exercise habits can be improved that I think my help will be worthwhile. The questions were good and easy to understand, I liked taking part in the interview" (female, aged 53)

Another elderly female mentioned the need to 'help' others who may be in a similar situation through research,

> "I like to help people, I am happy to reply to questions" (female, aged 68)

> "I like to help people on important projects, the results of this research might make people take note and understand why some people cannot afford to exercise though they want to. The government might make changes and allow people on low income and benefits to go to the gym for free or give them vouchers. The interview was excellent and the questions were very thorough" (male, aged 56)

What was surprising was the number of respondents who said they liked 'talking' about health issues. This is a good generic base on which to do further exploratory research around the health issues mentioned by respondents,

> "I like talking about health issues and if this research helps encourage people to take care of their health, exercise and eat right I will be proud to have helped out. The interview was enjoyable, the questions were good and detailed" (female, aged 49)

Another interviewee said,

> "I took part because this research could help people live more healthy lives. They might be taught how to eat and exercise to benefit their health" (female, aged 55)

A unique feature of the study was encouraging respondents to make comments about the interview process, indeed about the entire data collection phase. This is rarely done by researchers, but this important phase allows researchers to entertain new ideas about conducting research or, indeed, to maintain existing practices about the way research is conducted,

> "The questions were good but you did not ask me about smoking, that's a health issue for Asian people" (male, aged 54)

Ensuring that interviews are easy to understand, as well as the context of the research, cannot be understated for researchers. This is even more relevant because so many of the respondents in the present study had not been interviewed before. Equally, it helps if the respondents are talking about issues that are personally or directly relevant to them,

> "The questions were good and easy to understand. The interview was good, I liked talking about diet and exercise" (female, aged 57)

> "The questions were easy to understand, the interview was good. I enjoyed it" (female, aged 62)

Similarly,

> "I do not mind being interviewed, it is nice sometimes to talk about yourself, no one's asked me about my eating habits before. The questions were easy to understand and the interview was very good" (female, aged 54)

An interesting theme that arose from the interviews was that all respondents said they would participate in future health research if asked to do so,

> "Yes, of course, you can interview me about angina if you like" (male, aged 72)

Similarly, another respondent said,

> "I could help with research on high blood pressure" (woman, aged 61)

Most respondents had an interest in participating in health research; most often it was something personal to them, for example research on diet or exercise. The problem is that most people (especially minority groups) do not get the opportunity to be interviewed for research purposes because researchers often obtain their sample through official channels, such as community centres or through professional networks. This research was different since it did not obtain the sample by either of the two methods mentioned; this allowed those who had never been interviewed before to have an opportunity to express their views on health,

> "Yes, if I can help with health research, eating and exercise habits then I will do so" (female, aged 53)

> "If they are short and only a few questions I do not mind helping out. I hope other people get to know the importance of health and fitness. Without a person's health we cannot do much" (female, aged 68)

> "I am happy to participate in any health research, mental health research will be a good research to undertake" (male, aged 57)

Interest in research among respondents varied, for example, but what came out from the interviews was that research that is relevant to respondents' personal lives was always favoured, as well as helping others in similar situation,

> "Of course, you could interview me about my diet again if you like" (male, aged 56)

> "Yes, if you research on diet, I can help" (female, aged 51)

> "I could help with diet research" (female, aged 57)

> "Yes, health research about exercise or food" (female, aged 55)

Research has to be relevant to the individuals who take part in order to engage them in the research process; this, in turn, will help participants understand the purpose of the research. It is not always clear, by those taking part, how the research is designed to benefit them directly. At worse, some may feel that they are under scrutiny or examination and can lead them to become defensive and closed. Building trust between those conducting the research, and those who are researched, is crucial (as well those who are funding the research). This is more so when conducting research on a tightly-knit community, particularly on those groups that are often overlooked because of access problems (Din, 2006).

Dissemination

Participants will also want to know what will happen to the research once it has been completed, in terms of dissemination. Writing reports and presenting the findings at conferences is for academic purposes but, importantly, researchers need to ask the participants how they would like the research to be disseminated so it is presented in a helpful way to them. A good way of disseminating research is through workshops held in the local neighbourhood; again, community centres are ideal places because of the prominent location.

This should encourage the invitees to talk about the research and its implications. This also gives researchers the opportunities to explain the purpose of research and the possible benefits. The workshops are ideal places to get a flavour of how relevant the research was to those taking part (since there would be a gap between taking part and the dissemination activities), what worked well and, of course, what worked less well. Also, the probable benefit to participants who took part in the study.

If the participants have limited literacy skills, it is important to have available interpreters so the participants are in a position to contribute to the event in a constructive way. Disseminating research in this way allows a partnership to develop between researchers and the 'researched community'.

A word about the final report. I realise that there are cost implications in having the final report written in the community languages. However, if participants on the whole do not speak English, then the report should be made available in the main community languages and also in alternative formats, for example on audio tape so that individuals with limited language skills can listen to the findings (Din, 2006).

Accessing the over-researched? (Din, 2008)

There is some criticism from the Pakistani community that they have been over-researched in reference to health research. Often overlooked is the generic 'golden rule' of any research – it has to be both relevant and practical to participants so that they can engage with and find it beneficial to their everyday lives. Making research transparent and ensuring participants know what is involved are keys to accessing any community; equally, being part of the researched community can help, and living in the same neighbourhood as the respondents allows the researcher to be recognised (rather than being an 'outsider' who is only making contact with the community to conduct his/her fieldwork). There is an increasing need to conduct health research in Pakistan to find and quantify the health needs and outcomes of Pakistanis, both in Pakistan and also in the UK; equally, for service providers to be aware of social, cultural and religious influences on health behaviours, for example engaging in exercise activities and on diet and food choices.

Research methodologies have to adjust to the needs of the cohort. For example, it is often the case with young people (like most groups) that traditional research methods are inadequate in reaching the difficult 'minority within minority' groups. Both experience and, above all, knowing the community/groups well is essential. Bradford is an important geographical area where health research needs to be conducted, but this has to be both meaningful to those involved and carefully conducted. Central to the theme of this research was that it allows the voices of one minority ethnic community to be heard in the field of health research.

Textbooks on research methods often provide a prescriptive commentary on how to recruit participants; however, they sometimes overlook the difficulty in accessing and recruiting participants from a community setting. This is often due to lack of time spent in the community for purposes of data collection. The way to understand the struggles of collecting data in the community is to gain personal experience in the field, which can only be used over years as a junior researcher. Experience shows senior researchers rarely venture into the 'unknown', leaving it to juniors rarely passing on thoughts of wisdom of how to do this in a meaningful way. It becomes a survival tactic, for the field researcher goes out in the community looking for the minimum number of participants needed. Essentially, it's a numbers game.

What are lacking in literature are the strategies that are used in the real world to overcome problems of access and recruitment. The important thing to understand is that 'one size does not fit all' and different groups and communities require varied approaches. A textbook can point you in the right direction, but should really only be used as a stepping stone to devising a personal and individual recruitment strategy. Once you have this, you can revisit it and improve further.

The fruits of the labour are obvious: a well-prepared researcher will have confidence in presenting a carefully drafted recruitment plan. It shows foresight and creativity. Good researchers will see this as both a challenge and an opportunity to meet people rather than a chore. The advice I can offer to fieldworkers is perseverance and trial and error and, over time, you will hopefully learn new ways of engaging with groups and communities in a meaningful way.

CHAPTER FIVE

CONDUCTING RESEARCH IN PAKISTAN

> "People should contribute, we need to share knowledge and experience, past and present to build relations with doctors and researchers. We have people from all backgrounds so there are examples everywhere on every issue in health" (female, aged 68)

Sample

The sample takes into account the age, gender and socioeconomic background. A traditional sampling frame was not used; instead, opportunistic sampling, or the 'snowballing' technique, was used to recruit participants for the study. Community researchers and those with knowledge of the local area were asked for advice and support.

'Getting started'

The overarching aim for researchers is that research needs to be transparent and developed in a way that is easily understandable to lay people (for example, to non-English speakers) so they are better informed as to whether or not to participate in research. It is about making an informed decision. This is particularly relevant to Pakistan, where research is only beginning to come into the public domain. As discussed earlier, what made the difference was taking one's time to explain the research to individuals and the types of questions that would be asked; it was about reassuring individuals to the point they felt comfortable, which made recruitment easier. It was not unsurprising that most respondents in Mirpur had not participated in a research study previously,

> "It is the first time I have been interviewed by you" (male, aged 65)

> "This is the first time I have been interviewed before so it is good that you have started this research" (male, aged 63)

The initial thought was that male (rather than female) respondents would have participated in research previously. A point echoed by nearly all participants was,

> "I have never been interviewed before" (female, aged 62)

Whether they come from a community or health centre, or indeed through 'word of mouth', knowing the local community helps to make this process easier. The motto should be 'never miss an opportunity to recruit'. Recruitment is difficult even with years of experience; the best approach is to be proactive, creating a list of individuals and organisations that are willing to help.

Maintaining close links and rapport with these groups is essential during your data collection process and it can often prove fruitful. I remember the time when I was recruiting for a qualitative study examining biraderi (kin) support among the Pakistani population in West Yorkshire, UK, which included conducting one-to-one interviews followed by focus group interviews with members of the same family. Arranging focus group interviews is notoriously difficult, never mind arranging one at the home of the participant. The initial one-to-one interviews took place in the local community centre and, through this, a number of participants agreed for me to visit their house and conduct a follow-up focus group, which would include them (as parents), their siblings and extended kin, for example grandparents, living in the same household. Whether the participant says 'yes' or 'no' to a researcher depends upon the level of connection felt by the participant. They are deciding upon a number of factors, for example how you come across as an individual, whether there are any commonalities, such as shared religion and culture.

Perhaps the most important of these is language and whether they will be able to converse with you, not just in English but in the home language. What normally happens is that the language of the interview switches from English to the home language and then back to English. For example, whilst conducting an interview in, say, Mirpuri I find that key phrases or words are said in English. Being bilingual helps the communication process, thus ensuring the interview is fluid.

There was one exception in the form of an elderly gentleman who had been interviewed several times previously. He was a member of various societies in Mirpur and a respected elder (as discussed, often a first port of call for researchers looking for participants),

> "Many times I have been interviewed by different organisations" (male, aged 65)

Personally, elders in Pakistan are more than happy to help and access to organisations such madrasas and mosques are equally accessible. I suggest that, if you are conducting research in Pakistan, you take the elder with you to places where you would like to recruit from. The times I have done this I have learnt enormously; the 'elder' is able to reveal much more about the local population and groups residing in his/her district and changes over time than you will perhaps learn from reading a book. A nominal contribution towards travel costs and a meal is all that is required and always remember to acknowledge their contribution in the final report. It's a live commentary and a narrative about local people and places. As discussed earlier, by taking your time from getting from one place to another you learn about the surroundings; an added benefit is the attractive smells of street foods and the temptation for a very early lunch!

Respondents in Mirpur were positive about participating in research. There was an enormous amount of commonality among the responses, including feeling comfortable with the interviewer, or feeling 'happy' with the questions asked. For the researcher, this was about reflection, about what has worked and points to bear in mind for future reference, for example research that is relevant to people. The following respondent explains his initial hesitance but, as the interview went on, he 'felt comfortable',

> "This research is about health and this encouraged me to take part in this research. All the questions and the way you asked them were easy for me to understand. I felt comfortable about the interview, in the beginning I was hesitant but with time it was easy for me" (male, aged 65)

> "I felt comfortable about the interview and I felt relaxed during the interview and only in the beginning I was thinking perhaps it will be difficult and it was the first time" (male, aged 63)

The important thing to remember is that interviews are a two-way process allowing information to be shared; through this interchange is a raising of awareness among the respondents, as well a learning process for the interviewer. Much of this was a new experience for the respondents and they acknowledged this,

> "All types of research is informative and we do need someone to keep it this way. The questions are easy to understand, I did not have any problems during the interview" (male, aged 65)

The interview is not just about the researcher. The interview is a two-way process, the need for the researcher to ask a set number of questions, which answer the research question. It is also about the participant being able to 'receive something in return', in this case information about diet and exercise,

> "It also gave me a lot of knowledge about food and activities" (male, aged 65)

Researchers are in a good position to pass information on to participants especially, such as in this case, if the participant is unlikely to receive health information from any other source. Thus, the researcher is in a valuable position to help; attending with any available leaflets is a good way of information sharing with participants. The issue in Pakistan is the lack of community networks where people can simply 'pop in' for information. Instead, information is passed by 'word of mouth' from expert patients who have experienced a certain condition, for example patients suffering from diabetes. They can pass the knowledge to their friends and family about symptoms and treatments available. Literacy is another major problem, but we need to ensure the information is in an appropriate format, whether this is on an audio tape or DVD. The point to remember here is that 'one size does not fit all'; a close collaboration with individuals and families will lead to an improved outcome and the researcher will be in a better position to understand the needs of the participant.

Recruiting in Pakistan: from the community setting

Recruiting in Pakistan is, in my experience, wholly different from recruiting in the UK. As discussed earlier, participants from the Mirpur, Pakistan sample were recruited through using the 'snowballing' technique or 'word of mouth' with the help of key 'gatekeepers' (without whom my job would have been practically impossible). The main reason is that, although my parents were born and raised in Mirpur and emigrated to the UK during their 20s, and having traditional biraderi (kin) ties in Pakistan, I am considered a 'foreigner' (born and raised in the UK) or a 'vilayati' (an 'Englishman').

Mirpur (like most parts of Pakistan) does not have community centres or voluntary organisations (like in the British context), but it does have large numbers of masjids and madrassas which are found in all villages and towns across Pakistan that cater for the needs of people from different castes and sect groups (probably the two important ones), while other much smaller ones cater for particular biraderi (kin) groups. They are important places for meeting and general gossiping, given that Pakistan has a high rate of illiteracy, especially among the older groups, thus unable to read a newspaper. Information is gleaned through 'word of mouth'. Men (especially the older ones) meet daily, often after the daily prayers, to talk about anything interesting that is happening in their village or town, from the latest birth of a son to a couple that had been married for ten years, to the opening of a new shop in the mall, from the price of gold on the international market to the value of the rupee (compared to the British sterling). The atmosphere is often relaxed and comfortable, however there is little to do in terms of leisure activities; the more affluent ones may have a small screen television in one of the rooms. Popular TV programmes are the news, cricket and religious programmes

There are differences in terms of attendees; masjids are male-orientated, whereas madrassas allow females to attend and pray. They serve an important purpose, essentially a meeting place for women, young and old, to gather, normally in the evening. Otherwise, females would not normally be allowed to 'go out' like the men, for example to the bazaar to shop, so visiting a murdassa becomes an important outlet for females to gather.

I would assume that most leaders who run masjids and madrassas are forthcoming if researchers approached them with sensitivity and understanding and a thorough explanation of the research proposed. If the researcher is recruiting in Pakistan, I would suggest using a 'gatekeeper'.

It should not be an issue to recruit from masjids and madrassas. Muslims pray five times a day and, as a result, most masjid are full of worshippers around prayer times so there should be sufficient number of worshippers to recruit from. A point echoed earlier is to ensure, for example, information sheets have been translated, as a starting point in Urdu; also, however, information can be provided on a CD that is in a dialect, for example Mirpuri (the only proviso is that only some people will have access to a CD player). The ideal is to recruit through 'word of mouth' and in the dialect which the potential participants understand.

Health research in Pakistan

It is important to build rapport between the participants and the researcher, thus allowing for issues around diet and physical activity to be explored at some depth. Personally, I find that when the participant is 'happy' with the researcher, then this becomes a time for 'open dialogue', open-ended questions which allow for the participant to comment or narrate their story and for the interviewer to pick out key themes arising out of this communication, so as to delve further by means of using prompts. It is a job of the researcher (and a skilful task) to help navigate the discussion guide, carefully helping the participant to concentrate on the important questions on the discussion guide. Although most researchers will tell you that 'time is of the essence' and the need for you to get through the discussion guide 'as quickly as possible', I find that most people (especially in Pakistan) value the opportunity to have a discussion with someone of a different background to theirs, especially someone from overseas.

This was particularly important in a country like Pakistan, which needs to develop a strong research base in order to cater for the needs of its people and in order to introduce health policies and measure outcomes in the future,

> "If someone comes to me for an interview regarding health research I will definitely participate. Health research about exercise or on any type of diseases I will participate because this way I will be more aware about health matters" (male, aged 65)

> "I will participate in all types of health research and which will make us aware about our food choices and that fight against diseases" (male, aged 63)

> "It is important for everyone to participate in all types of research because we would get more awareness through such types of research. There should be a special programme to make people aware in this way, also people could be encouraged to participate in health research" (male, aged 65)

Again, the will to participate in order to raise awareness was clear among the respondents. It was an individual's 'duty as a good citizen' to promote in research,

> "I will definitely participate in all types of research because in this way we will do our duty as a good citizen and we will get information as well" (male, aged 65)

Others mentioned that researchers should help people to learn about 'research' and its importance. A point made earlier was that researchers need to sell research to communities in a way that is positive; it is equally paramount that participating individuals realise the wider benefits that it can bring about, for example informing policy,

> "People should be educated to know about the importance of research" (male, aged 65)

> "There should be more awareness about doing interviews for research, especially these kinds of interviews as they play an important role in changing their life and lifestyle" (female, aged 65)

One participant suggested that researchers could arrange programmes to raise awareness,

> "It is important for everyone to participate in health research because they can be aware about health. We should arrange special programmes so that people can be encouraged to participate in health research" (male, aged 63)

The majority of the Mirpur sample said they would like the results to be disseminated on an audio tape and in an appropriate language,

> "I would like the result of this research disseminated through audio tape or written so it is easy for me to understand and also that it is in my own language" (male, aged 65)

> "The results of this research should be disseminated either as written or audio tape or through conference" (male, aged 65)

Another elderly male mentioned that he would like to attend a conference to find out about the results of the research studies,

> "Results of this research should be disseminated by conference because it would be easy for me or it should be on audio tape" (male, aged 63)

CHAPTER SIX

DIETARY HABITS IN PAKISTAN

> "It is not good here (Mirpur) because nowadays people are very lazy because people now mostly depend upon takeaways instead of eating fresh food" (female, aged 61)

Like in all countries, food consumption is dependent upon family income. There is no welfare support like we have in the UK. However, Pakistan has a system of Zakat (charity) where a small amount of money is distributed to the very poorest of families, for example to widows or those families where the father or both parents have died. However, some affluent families give financial and other assistance to poorer families in their neighbourhood; for example, it is not uncommon to give unwanted items of clothing or pay for food, and some private schools provide subsidised free school places to children whose parents are unable to afford school fees.

Pakistan is primarily a third world country and the majority of Pakistanis live below the poverty line, which impacts their buying power. Most Pakistani families live 'day by day' and their diet varies considerably; for example, if the father works on a regular basis then the family can afford to buy sufficient food to feed the family. Given that the family size is much larger (when compared to European families), many families have extended family members living in the same household and need to support them, for example, in-laws, grandparents and unmarried uncles and aunts. This obviously has a knock-on effect (and an increased cost) in the number of mouths to feed.

In most 'Asian' cultures, eating food is a communal event, for example during weddings, birthdays and during Ramadan and Eid. During my visit to Pakistan in 2006, I noticed that, nearly everywhere you looked, food was either being prepared or being sold to consumers. Freshly-fried savouries were a favourite among the shoppers as was fresh produce grown by local farmers.

A particularly important time for celebration for biraderi (kin) members is when relatives arrive from the UK. Various dishes are prepared and family and biraderi members gather to meet their overseas friends. It is a joyous occasion, but also a time to 'show' their status in the community by inviting as many people as they can to dinner. Relatives will always bring sweetmeat when they visit. Typically, dinner will be served at 8pm and guests will continue to consume the various dishes late into the night.

Typically during a communal gathering it is not uncommon to see the following foods being served. For example, the starter will include: pakora, onion bhajis, samosas, seekh kebabs and grilled lamb chops. The main meal often include the following: a meat curry (chicken, lamb), a vegetable curry (cauliflower and potato, spinach and potato), a mixed meat and vegetable curry (chicken and cauliflower) and a lentil curry (for example, chickpeas) served with fresh roti and naans. This is followed by tea and sweet desserts: flooda, Asian sweets and ice cream. Drinks include mango lassi, sweet lassi and fizzy drinks. Salad is also served which includes tomatoes, onions, horseradish and iceberg lettuce. Fruit includes watermelon, oranges, apples, bananas and strawberries. It is interesting to note that all the food served is seasonal and fresh and much of this is organic or home-grown.

It is important to remember that access to foods depends upon the financial position of the family. Some families in Pakistan can purchase 'what they like', for example meat, while most families in Pakistan rely on the basic essentials to survive. Meat is considered as a luxury commodity only to be consumed on special occasions, for example on Eid (most families will save for a month to have this on their dinner plate).

Most Pakistanis live below the poverty line and typically the family household in Pakistan includes the parents, siblings, married siblings, and grandparents (and may also include uncles and aunts). The family household is typically extended and this is true of many Pakistani families residing in the UK. Depending upon the social and economic status, most families find the household budget is stretched with little 'left over' for emergencies, such as medical bills.

Mirpur is considered as an affluent area (this is particularly true, as remittances are sent by families from the UK to relatives in Pakistan) and these families can maintain some level of adequate living. However, most families do not have any financial support or help and are completely self-reliant. This has an enormous knock-on effect upon families, for example most can only afford to give their children primary education, while very little if anything is spent on social activities. In fact, most are unable to afford adequate clothing. A typical trait of Pakistani families is an early marriage among both genders; upon marriage, the daughter will move in with her in-laws, whereas the son will remain in the family household.

Society in Pakistan is divided along the lines of caste (see Din, 2006). The highest caste in Pakistan are the Rajahs and the Jats, who are the 'landed gentry' and who own most of the land in Pakistan. They are also successful business people running their own private hospitals, medical centres and large shopping malls. The rent from the latter can amount to millions of rupees a month.

The next most affluent groups are the Bhengse, who are middle income landowners. They will own land and usually grow fruit and vegetables to sell to local people in their village and town. Most will also own medium-sized shopping malls or shops in Plazas to subsidise their income. A number of them own their own primary (and secondary) schools attended by up to several hundred local children, all charging anything up to 1500 rupees (approximately £10) a month.

These are followed by the Morchis, who are the shoesmiths. Others who are part of this caste include silversmiths and horsesmiths. These groups are trained to do specific tasks that have been handed down through generations, for example the shoesmith will make and repair shoes. In recent years, the shoesmith has been repairing shoes rather than making them due to the ready-made market; shoes are arriving from overseas to cater for the needs of the population as a result of an increase in financial resources.

Those with the least amount of income are the day labourers who work on a daily rate, typically around 700 rupees (approx. £5). Their work is invariably manual and varied; for example, one day they could be laying the foundations for a road and the next they could be decorating a house. They work anything between 12 to 16 hours a day; it is physically hard work and, during the hot, scorching summer months of Pakistan, only the fittest and healthiest of men work. Thus, no income is generated and most men are unable to even provide the minimal amount of food on the table.

During times of austerity and financial hardship, I found that in many households across Pakistan women become the family's saviour, as well as doing the household chores, looking after the children and extended family members. The wife will engage in working from home and, if they have an older daughter, they too will help their mother. Typical types of work engaged is seamstress work or making savouries to sell in the bazaar.

Typically, the married woman's day will be as follows. Once all the daily household chores are completed, for example making breakfast, cleaning the house, etc., the wife will start cutting the cloth and start sewing the material. For each completed suit, she will receive anything between 400 to 800 rupees (depending upon the difficulty and additional sewing she may have to do). However, sewing men's suits can earn twice as much, around 1500 rupees. This is a back-breaking exercise; most women find they spend anything up to 10 hours or more a day sewing. Through this, they essentially prevent the family from becoming destitute, especially where the husband is unable to work or has died. It is important to remember that, for most women, this is a struggle they endure on a daily basis.

Typical day's cooking in Mirpur

The mother usually gets up at 6am and starts with some of her daily chores, for example sweeping the main foyer or doing the washing. Few households in Pakistan can afford a washing machine, thus it is a chore done by hand, often using soap and cold water from a storage tank or, if they are fortunate, from a well dug in the garden. Since the water storage tank has to be filled from a mobile tanker, they charge anything up to 15,000 rupees depending upon the number of litres of water required. Fresh water in Pakistan is expensive.

Breakfast

Typically, most Pakistani families will have their breakfast at 7am; the husband normally leaves for work about this time in the summer. The wife prepares and cooks breakfast for all the family. For many of the poorer families in Pakistan, breakfast will comprise roti and curry, something wholesome to get through to lunch time (but much of this depends upon the financial resources of the family). However, families with higher incomes will have eggs, toast, cereal, freshly-baked biscuits and cakes from the local bakery, orange juice and milk. This is a reflection of the family's economic fortune.

Lunchtime

As soon as the breakfast is served, the mother starts preparing for lunch, and fresh ingredients need to be bought from the bazaar (especially in the summer months to ensure they are fresh). This is usually the job of the elder son (older, unmarried girls rarely venture to the bazaar) as it is a male-dominated space. He will be given money by the mother and it is his job to make sure that he buys all the ingredients for the lunchtime meal. This is normally done by 10am. The method of cooking varies; some families cook on the open fire (often, locals provide free wood) as they are unable to afford the luxury of a gas cooker. Lunchtime is around 1pm and most families will have roti and curry (this is normally vegetable or lentil curry) served with side salads and lassi. Again, the meals are filling in order to get through the day because the main meal will not be served until late evening.

Main evening meal

The main evening meal is around 10pm, when the husband returns home from a long day's work. It is the main meal of the day and all the family members gather to eat as well as discuss family business. Again, the main meal consists of roti and curry (normally meat or chicken). For others less affluent, it may be vegetable or lentil curry. The meal is followed by tea and fresh cakes and biscuits from the local bakery.

Do you think you eat healthily?

What comes through strongly in the interviews is that those individuals and families with financial resources could afford to eat healthily. The difference between the lifestyle of affluent groups and poorer families becomes apparent through these interviews. We explore the issue of accessibility of different foods, but also the participants' knowledge of different foods, what is good and what is bad for their body and what is a balanced diet.

For the more affluent participants, the importance of trying to eat healthily is important, as is a diet that is varied and balanced. Given their busy lifestyle, the more affluent families often employ a cook or a chef to prepare their meals, normally paying 5,000 rupees a month. This makes it easier to prepare fresh, wholesome and balanced meals, especially the main evening meal, where observational work suggests that most calories are consumed. They tend to prepare less fried foods, replacing them with healthier options, for example grilling the food instead.

It is interesting to note that, in Western countries, food is served as a 'portion', for example a slice of meat with a portion of vegetables. However, in the Pakistani context, this is irrelevant, as the 'size' of the meal is large. The plate size has an important influence; simply, the bigger the plate the bigger the portion. Food is served to the rim and loaded on top; it's a cultural trait which represents the fact that those enjoying the meal will leave the table completely full. Culturally, smaller plates are a poor reflection on the host family since they denote the family as being 'poor'.

Typically, the individual will consume a starter, for example pakoras, followed by a main meal, usually around 4pm, with a meat or vegetable dish (again, dependent upon the affordability of the individual/family). The desire to eat healthily runs throughout the interviews,

> "I try to eat healthily and so I eat all types of food so I feel myself as being healthy" (male, aged 65)

The important thing for respondents was to try and eat as healthily as possible and keep to a balanced diet. The important thing was that most respondents understood the importance of keeping to a balanced diet, even though at times they struggled and gave into temptation of their favourite high-calorie foods,

> "I eat healthy food I try my best to eat healthily and the food you eat should be balanced" (male, aged 65)

There were differences between the social groups, where the more affluent families enjoyed a much more varied diet. As mentioned above, employing a chef meant that he/she was in charge of preparing low calorie meals to suit the requirements of the family.

Typical of affluent households in Mirpur, the chef would prepare two main dishes a day, a meat dish and a vegetable dish, and would use the minimum amount of oil. This also meant they were likely to maintain a healthy weight and less likely to snack between meals,

> "I eat healthily, I take care in what I eat but I like all types of food" (male, aged 60)

By contrast, the majority of families on very limited income would have 'what they could afford'. For example, the majority of the day labourers will have consumed very simple foods (bearing in mind that most labourers earn around 700 rupees a day,

> "I am a healthy man because I like to eat very simple foods" (male, aged 63)

In reality, the main meal of the day for the poorer families would be a 'one course meal', comprising a simple dish such as potato curry with the minimum of ingredients and spices added to enhance the flavour and to make it more palatable. For others who are even less fortunate, they will prepare watery mint chutney and have this with a roti.

Pakistan is a developing country and, although Mirpur has millions of pounds of remittances sent to the district by overseas patrons, most of the population largely remains poor, living 'day to day' and often below the breadline. The lack of employment opportunities is a real challenge. So, although some medium-sized businesses operate in Mirpur, the vast majority are small, family-run businesses employing one or two people. They are the fortunate ones who probably can just about afford to get by on a minimum wage. As a result of a lack of major employers in the district, much of the population is unemployed; even those with some qualifications find it very difficult to secure a job. Governmental jobs (when they become available) are prized since they have reasonably good pay, conditions and benefits such as access to healthcare.

The poorest of the day labourers are entirely dependent upon the work available to them locally. Typically, major cities such as Mirpur will have plenty of labouring employment available, whereas smaller, outlying villages will have very few daily opportunities available. Travelling between towns and cities to find work is common and, as mentioned earlier, the work is poorly paid and often seasonal.

For most people in Mirpur, aspirations are 'realistic'. The overriding goal for most Pakistanis is to survive and 'get by' as best they can and, at the same time, fulfil cultural aspirations such as getting married and starting a family. This is an area where cultural traditions help poorer families; for example, living together in an extended family ensures that everyone sticks together and helps each other. Those who are fortunate enough to have a job help to pay for food and services for the whole family. In this way, no-one in the family is left behind and everyone shares all they have. However, this type of living has obvious economic and social advantages. It can also act as a basis for tension between family members and cause economic strain on the already tight finances of the family, for example if a family member requires on-going medical treatment.

Do you know what a balanced diet is?

Most participants interviewed for this book acknowledged the importance of maintaining a balanced diet; for example, they all accepted that consuming fried foods twice a day was not 'healthy' (although a number of them did actually have fried foods). They did so because fried foods such as pakoras and samosas were viewed as being 'filling' and would keep them going through the day, especially in the case of a day labourer working on a 12-hour shift, which was hard, and the way to get through the day was to make sure they had enough food. However, what was interesting to note was that children were also served fried foods at breakfast and before they went to school, again to keep them from being hungry whilst at school. Mobile caterers are often seen outside schools serving fried foods to schoolchildren, and fried foods are much cheaper when compared to the healthier options. They also serve fizzy drinks, sweets and chocolates, while the 'best sellers' in the hot summer months are kulfi (ice cream) and flooda (very sweet dessert).

When asked the question 'do you know what a balanced diet is?' common responses among families on limited incomes was that they had little knowledge about what a 'balanced' diet is,

> "I do not have the knowledge of what a balanced diet is" (female, aged 65)

Further, for some of these families, meals were 'set', meaning that they had the same or similar foods each and every day with little financial scope for variation in their diet,

> "I don't have much knowledge about what a balanced diet is. Traditionally we have a set meal, it's like a schedule like what we are going to eat today and what we will eat tomorrow" (female, aged 60)

Again, 'poor' families were considerably restricted in their purchasing power of available foods. They tended to purchase foods from street traders which are generally cheaper (because of lower overheads and rents), thus are in a position to pass savings onto the customer. Compare this to shops that are located in one of the big shopping malls; they sell foods at a higher price not only because of higher business rents, but because they generally sell higher-quality produce. They meet the particular demands of overseas Pakistanis who are visiting Pakistan and are in search of quality foods. These are the shopping places of choice for affluent families, whereas the poorer families again echo their present predicament,

> "I do not know what a balanced diet is, we only eat such foods which we can afford because I belong to a poor family" (male, aged 63)

Again,

> "I eat vegetables and whatever is available in the market or what is affordable to us, it is bad we do not eat regularly what we would like to eat. It is not our choice in terms of what we eat" (male, aged 63)

It was interesting to note how 'knowledge' of a balanced diet was shared, particularly among kin members. Those who had been fortunate enough to spend time overseas, for example in the UK, learnt about food and the impact poor food choices can have on the body. They learnt this through health messages and publications, but also through examples of kin members who had long-term conditions such as diabetes and coronary heart disease, which are prevalent among South Asian populations. They realised that one has to make careful food choices, otherwise there is the very real possibility of the negative impact this can have later. At the same time, the following respondent observes that people in Pakistan do not have 'knowledge' about what a balanced diet is, however his stay in England has been a learning experience,

> "I have spent my life abroad (England) so I have some knowledge about what a balanced diet is, otherwise people here (Pakistan) have no knowledge about what a balanced diet is" (male, aged 62)

This is understandable given the rates of illiteracy in Pakistan, particularly among the females, older people and those living in remote areas of the district. Getting the health message across to different populations about eating healthily and exercising is an uphill challenge for most health professionals, irrespective of the country, but particularly for developing countries where financial resources are limited. Having locally-trained professionals who are in a position to understand local customs and norms would, I imagine, be the best placed people to help put health messages across. Another respondent had extensive knowledge about healthy eating, coming as he was from an affluent background and educated to a degree level. He explained about the essentials of consuming vitamins,

> "I know what a balanced diet is, it is equal proportion of all vitamins essential to your body" (male, aged 65)

Do you worry about what you are eating?

During the next discussion, respondents were asked whether they worry about what they eat. This led to an interesting discussion with participants allowing the researcher to examine food choices of participants. The importance of building rapport with respondents comes into its own when they feel comfortable about discussing the subject matter in an open manner, and setting the scene is important. The shift between generations is particularly worth noting, as the following respondent explains when he mentions the younger generation enjoy takeaway foods, which are high in calories,

> "I try to avoid such types of food like fizzy drinks and takeaways, but the younger generation are now depending upon such types of foods" (male, aged 65)

Where it was easier for the older generations to avoid such foods as fizzy drinks and takeaways, the younger generations are beginning to enjoy a different palate. It also represents the import of foreign foods and flavours; where once Mirpuris had samosas and pakoras, they are now enjoying flavours from around the world from pizzas and pasta to fish and chips. It is evident among those who can afford these foods that a globalisation of taste buds has taken hold of young Pakistanis and this will only increase as more and more individuals increase their income.

The consumption of Western foods is seen as a status symbol and a break from traditions. To be seen in a takeaway outlet demonstrates wealth and affluence. Those with money want to be seen in a fast food outlet.

Bearing in mind a day labourer earns about 700 rupees, the following are prices for takeaway foods in Mirpur. As you can see, the following foods are out of reach of most people in Mirpur. Typically, a 12" pizza costs 600 rupees, a piri piri chicken meal that includes fries and a drink costs 1000 rupees, a burger meal again with fries and a drink costs 600 rupees, large fish and chips costs 1200 rupees, a meal for two Western-style chicken and chips with a drink costs 600 rupees. There has been an increase in 'all you can eat' food outlets in Mirpur, Rawalpindi and Islamabad. For example, 'all you can eat' including fizzy drinks in a pizzeria in Mirpur costs 1200 rupees. For the majority of Pakistanis, and because of lack of money, they have no choice but to continue eating simple foods prepared at home,

> "I am not worried about eating fatty foods, fizzy drinks or takeaways because we cannot afford to so we eat simple food (desi)" (male, aged 63)

Fast foods for the majority are seen as being 'luxury' foods. Another respondent echoed the cooking habits of the majority,

> "We prepare our food at home and we know that we should eat all things like vegetables, pulses and meat" (female, aged 65)

Cultural traditions dictate that mothers teach the daughters to cook, usually from the age of about eight. The mother allows her daughter to cut vegetables and lay out the ingredients for the mother to start preparing the curry dish. It is worth remembering that there is no 'trial and error', as one learns to cook properly the first time, given the expense of ingredients. Later, as the daughter becomes confident in the kitchen, she is introduced to preparing the dish, usually inexpensive pulses and lentils at first since, if anything goes wrong, then there is no great loss. Later, the daughter is allowed to prepare meat and chicken dishes, which are the most expensive. By the time their daughter reaches adulthood, much of the cooking will be done by her; the mother will devote her time to younger siblings, or she may be engaged in domestic labour or working from home, usually as a seamstress.

The shift from a basic diet to incorporating different foods is obvious, as is the worry among some older people that there is an on-going strong influence of fast foods. Such foods are viewed by many older people as being lacking in thakath ('strength'), meaning they are lacking in essential vitamins. They are therefore avoided by the old, but the young desire such foods,

> "I try to avoid such types of food but I worry about our younger generation, they are now starting to eat more takeaways, cakes and drink fizzy drinks" (male, aged 60)

Similarly, another older respondent echoes the importance of eating desi (organic) foods and the need to avoid fizzy drinks containing high amounts of sugar,

> "I worry about the food I am eating. I try my best to eat pure desi food (organic) and try to avoid fizzy drinks and cakes" (male, aged 65)

Older Pakistanis had grown up on staple foods such as lentils, pulses, chicken, fruits and vegetables. Many, when introduced to Western foods, rejected them on the basis of not being able to digest such foods. Beef burgers and pizzas were seen as foreign foods consumed by Western people and, when introduced in Pakistan, they largely avoided them, instead staying with traditional foods. A growing minority, however, have taken a liking to Western foods and enjoy such foods as much as their young. This also represents a shift in identity as it is not just about food consumption, but being a global consumer.

Knowing how much one weighs

With a growing obesity epidemic, especially in the developed world, governments are increasingly under a financial strain to meet the health needs of patients who are suffering from obesity-related conditions. As obesity rates rise, so too have health budgets; this is particularly a problem for developing countries like Pakistan, who are struggling to meet the health needs of all sections of its population.

Most participants said they do not weigh themselves on a regular basis. In fact, most did not know exactly how much they weigh. Just to clarify, observational data suggested that most households visited did not own a weighing scale of their own, nor did they have access to one; they simply couldn't afford one. In some cases, there was no need to own one because visually they looked either underweight or 'just about right'. However, in cases where an increase in weight was becoming an issue, interestingly it was left to friends and family members to let the individual know if they had put on weight and perhaps needed to shed a few pounds. It was a public discussion rarely taken as a personal offence. This had positive outcomes, for some were family members who acted as a control mechanism, thus ensuring alarm bells would sound if an individual was overeating.

Most were weighed at the doctor's surgery or at the health clinic – if they could afford the clinic fees, that is. Again, affordability was an issue and especially important if the patient was suffering from type 2 diabetes, in which case the need to maintain a healthy weight was paramount. In this regard, a day labourer responded by saying (and this was similarly echoed by many others),

> "No, I am not watchful about my weight. I do not know how much I weigh. I think my weight is alright so I would not like to lose or gain any weight. I cannot remember when I weighed myself last" (male, aged 65)

Although most participants did not know exactly how much they weighed, they had an instinctive 'feel' about whether their weight was 'alright'. Others admitted they never have weighed themselves,

> "I do not know how much I weigh. I have never weighed myself and I can only guess about my weight" (male, aged 63)

For the older generation, 'guessing' one's weight was common among family members. It was also common for participants from this sample to 'give up' food or 'skip' a meal to ensure young grandchildren had a 'proper' meal. This was particularly common among participants with very limited incomes. Typically, foods which would be given up for grandchildren were desserts, cakes and biscuits. In the case of guests invited for an evening meal, immediate family members would be served last; this was to ensure that guests were fully fed first, then children would be fed, followed by parents and, lastly, grandparents.

Data from my previous study, which examined diet and physical activity among older Pakistanis in Bradford, revealed the extent of keeping a careful eye on one's weight. The constant keeping track of one's weight was regularly done, more so if one was suffering from diabetes or high blood pressure. This was important because of the long-term debilitating consequences of diabetes,

> "I am watchful about my weight and I regularly weigh myself. I know how much I weigh since I have maintained my weight, since I weigh myself every two or three days" (male, aged 65)

> "I am watchful about my weight because I regularly weigh myself and I know how much I weigh" (male, aged 60)

Taking a personal case study, most of my relatives had suffered or suffer from diabetes. It is so common that it is almost considered as being 'normal' to have the condition, especially in later life. Further, coronary heart disease and high blood pressure are equally present among Pakistanis. At the same time, seeing relatives suffer from diabetes-related conditions such as amputations has been common over the years, as is those who had or are currently having dialysis. Dialysis is a long-term condition and a few of my relatives have been fortunate enough to have received a kidney transplant; most, however, have died waiting for a suitable donor. For most struggling with their weight (certainly in their adulthood), all the interventions by health professionals have seemed to all but fail, such as learning self-control.

Stigma can act as control mechanism for the individual, however this also seems to have failed. Family, friends and the community all try to play a positive role in helping the individual control their weight. Most, I have to say, are positive and constructive comments to aid the individual but, again, like the health messages, they have failed.

Being overweight or obese has a knock-on effect on family life (as discussed in existing literature). Individuals often retreat from public and also their family life. This lack of engagement has also had an adverse effect on the individual, who often fails to maintain a happy home life and, if they are trying to start a life, this can also reduce their chances due to their weight. Particularly poignant are those parents who have young siblings, as their failure to engage in sports activities or other recreational activities can lead to all but absent parents.

Retreating from family life within the Pakistani community is all but unheard of. In Pakistan, family functions such as births, deaths and marriages are attended by all family members, with no exceptions (apart from those who are bedridden). It is an expectation and a public display of affiliation and loyalty to the kin network. Grandparents and elders are expected to attend all functions, whatever their other commitments. Functions are essentially about being able to transmit the biraderi's norms, values and attitudes to their young, who will be present. One important way of transmitting stories of the old is through storytelling; stories that recapture hardships and heroics of the forefathers and how they were able to come through times of need and survive, are told. Stories of hope are revered and, through the narrative, the elders can once again relive and feel wanted. In a society which still largely holds enormous respect and loyalty towards older relatives, many younger people listen attentively. The hope for the older generations is that their stories will live on and be re-told to future generations.

It is not easy to 'hide away' from public life. The pressures are enormous and it is something that is wholly unsustainable over a period of time. This is unlike cases of morbidly obese people in Western countries, who at times have disappeared in complete seclusion, some stuck in their homes as prisoners, others rarely venturing out of their bedroom, never mind their house, completely reliant on their spouse, sibling or their carer. Again, general observations suggest that the pressure for obese Pakistanis is such that they maintain a certain amount of 'normality' and, if they are able to, walk.

At the same time, seeing the struggle on the part of relatives and family members to curb their eating habits is a daily struggle. Advice and counselling from health professionals has, on the whole, been ignored. Health messages, irrespective of format, also have been ignored by patients who are struggling to keep the condition under control.

Personal space is not an issue in Pakistan as it is in most Western countries, where houses are generally small (cottage, terrace, semi-detached houses) when compared to the amount of space available to the individual in Pakistan, where houses are large. The individual buys land – a small-size plot of land is called a marla, a large plot is called kanal – and then they plan, design and construct the house. It is not uncommon for the lounge and reception rooms to be 30-foot long and the bedrooms to be 20-foot long. The height of the door frame is similar to that of the British, but the width of the doors is generally wider to allow easier delivery of furniture into the house. Doors are wider because, in Pakistan, furniture is often handmade and comes ready assembled.

Observation in Pakistan provided useful insight into the eating behaviour of families, particularly when weight gain is of concern. Among the Mirpuris, it was noted that weight increased among young people (aged 14-24) and those in their 50s. This was noticeable among both males and females. Talking to older people suggests that, when they get older, they start to reduce their level and intensity of work (especially if they have been engaged in manual work during their adult life). Reasons given included that they didn't 'feel as strong' as when they were younger, although they acknowledged that they need to carry on working as long as possible to keep supporting the family. 'Worries' about the future prospects of their immediate family, the lack of income, ill health and finding suitable marriage partners for their marriageable age children were further reasons that led them to eating more.

There are a number of social pressures that contribute towards individuals relying on food as a 'comfort'. They also contribute towards mental health and depression. The issue that creates the most pressure on parents and families in Pakistan (and the UK) is marriage. The age of marriage in Pakistan is much younger than in the UK; typically, a daughter would be married by the age of 20 (those from poorer backgrounds). Boys have several more years of independence, for the fact that they will remain in the family home; sons also act as the male breadwinner (taking over the role from the father). It is the difficulty of finding a suitable marriage partner for the daughter that can act as a trigger for depression for parents (having seen this in many Pakistani families, see Din 2006, Cullingford and Din, 2000). There are often conflicts between kin members, with the desire to marry their daughter among cousins at the same time to break away from traditions of forefathers.

Do you look at the contents of the food?

A number of participants (those who were literate) said that they read the content of the foods they were purchasing. This applied to Western foods, for example when purchasing cereals, biscuits, sweets and cakes.

> "I think foods are clear to read in terms of their fat contents except some foods like some local products, but we try to use all real products or well-known products, whether they are national or international" (male, aged 60)

Similarly, another respondent said,

> "I think the food contents are clear to understand and read in terms of their fats or calories to some extent" (male, aged 65)

Changing labels on packages is a way forward,

> "I only look at the pictures on the tins or box when I go shopping with my friend, which is not that often. When I see a picture of a cake I think 'yes' that is nice I will buy it. I do sometimes ask the assistants if this is good or bad for me to eat. I can read Urdu, if the packaging was changed that would be good" (female, aged 68)

The following respondent highlighted the 'small writing' on food products was difficult to read, as poor eyesight was a major factor,

> "The contents of the foods are clear to understand in terms of their contents except some products, where they are written in small writing" (male, aged 65)

What is interesting is the confidence expressed by the above respondents when they are able to read the 'fats or calories' of foods they consume. Again, it is the most literate of respondents who are in a position to make such an informed choice. Decisions about food choice among those with limited language skills in English and Urdu are dependent upon literate friends and family.

One of the reasons why participants looked at the contents was to see if the product contained any animal fats, especially any non-halal ingredients. Pakistan is a Muslim country and products containing animal products would not be sold in Pakistan; despite this, there was still a tendency to look at the ingredients. It also shows that customers were becoming more knowledgeable about what they were purchasing. It must be noted that these participants were the exceptions rather than the norm. The majority of ordinary Pakistanis did not have the income to be able to afford Western foods. One participant said,

> "I look at the contents of the food" (male, aged 65)

Suffering from a food allergy also led to customers to check the content of the food. Again, foreign foods were quoted, including milk products. The ability to read English and the knowledge to understand the calorific information meant that only a small number of consumers could engage in this activity. For most others, the following were expressed,

> "I do not look at the contents of food, we have no concept about it whether we should look or not" (male, aged 63)

Similarly, another respondent said,

> "We have no concept of looking at the contents of food, very rarely we look at the contents" (female, aged 61)

This is similar to the findings of my earlier work on the diet of Pakistanis in Bradford,

> "I do not look at the contents of foods in terms of their calories and fat" (male, aged 65)

Again,

> "We do not look at the contents of the food and we do not have such information either or indeed what we should be looking for" (female, aged 60)

Another respondent went on to explain that Pakistani families eat fresh foods rather than packed foods,

> "We don't look at the contents of the food because mostly we buy fresh food and not packed foods" (female, aged 65)

In my experience, I have never heard of a Pakistani family serving a readymade meal to guests or even family. Although there are numerous vegetarian and meat dishes on the market, it would be 'unusual' for a Pakistani to purchase one in the UK and even rarer in Pakistan. However, there is generational change occurring among Pakistani families, both in the UK and Pakistan. The frozen food market has exploded, selling products such as frozen samosas, seekh kebabs, meat burgers, chicken burgers and vegetable rolls among the favourites. Such foods would normally take a lot of preparation time, especially when the 'family' is invited.

A typical large family get-together in Bradford would mean inviting around 30 to 40 family members, and it would not be uncommon to serve 150 samosas and 200 seekh kebabs, for example. Other 'homemade' foods might include 80 chicken tikkas, 10 kilos of pakoras, meat curry (5 kilos of meat), chicken curry (15 kilos of chicken), 20 kilos of pilau rice (including meat), 8 kilos of sweet rice, 10 kilos of carrot dessert, 100 rotis and 20 2.5 litre bottles of fizzy drinks.

It is interesting to point out that, culturally, it is difficult for individuals to control their diet where 'eating' is seen as a communal activity. Everyone is encouraged to eat and everyone who can eat eats, and all the dishes on the table are tried. So, when three or four dishes are served with several starters and desserts to follow, one can imagine how this can lead to overeating. No-one is encouraged to eat in moderation, or leave the table feeling that they could have had another samosa or a pakora. The more one eats, the happier the host. Since most of the food is cooked fresh, the understanding is food that is on the table is to be consumed, since the idea of reheating food the following day is unusual, certainly in Pakistan. With few families being able to afford a fridge or a freezer, a curry dish is consumed at one sitting.

Leaving the table prematurely, and certainly before trying all the dishes, can be seen as being 'disrespectful' to the host. The cultural etiquette is for everyone to sit together and to go through all the dishes.

Most Pakistanis who immigrated to the UK came from poor rural backgrounds and most struggled to feed their family. A particularly difficult time for millions of Pakistanis was the period after Independence in 1947, when millions of Muslims were uprooted to make their homes in the newly-formed Pakistan. Poverty on all sides was rife, with many struggling to survive from day to day and not knowing where the next meal would be coming from, or where they would settle. My parents, like the majority of Mirpuris who came to the UK, settled in Mirpur, quickly establishing small communities based on kin membership. The struggle was collective and what little they had was shared equally amongst the 'family'. Later, poverty was a key factor that encouraged Pakistanis to emigrate to the UK when the opportunity arose (discussed earlier).

After Independence, flour was in short supply and considered by many as 'gold dust'. The wealth of the family was measured by the quantity of flour (and other basics they were able to afford, the prized foods being salt, sugar, tea, chillies, vegetable ghee) they had in their kitchen. Those fortunate enough to afford tea had it black, as milk was very scarce. Instead, families (again, if they were able to afford it) had cardamon in their tea to give some flavour.

Very few families could afford to invite dinner guests. The majority relied on what they could muster; it was not uncommon to go unfed for days. The major problem was employment in the region, as very few had 'jobs'. Much of the employment was based on need, for example a shoesmith or blacksmith would have work coming in and were usually paid with 'food' (usually tea, sugar or flour) instead of cash. Enormous improvement was seen during the 1970s, especially with remittances sent to relatives left behind in Mirpur.

As things improved and finances become easier, Pakistanis began to enjoy all sorts of foods. Meat and chicken had always been prized because of the expense, now most are able to have them on a weekly basis in Mirpur. The affordability of food has led to Pakistanis eating 'as and when' and there is always a reason to celebrate! For example, the Month of Fasting, Eid, while births and marriages are celebrated at family get-togethers.

For Pakistanis arriving in the UK, they quickly became able to afford what they wanted to consume. Those who managed to save money in the early days set up corner shops selling staple Halal foods, while those who owned butcher shops were particularly successful in their enterprises. This financial success equated to a substantial increase in 'izzat' (honour, status) of the family, both here in the UK and also in Pakistan. Izzat was and is still 'prized' and for individuals to be respected by their fellow kinfolk.

Calories consumed

Although there was general knowledge about food content, for example the main ingredients in a product, this did not equally apply to the amount of calories within foods,

> "I have no knowledge about calories" (female, aged 61)

Typically, most respondents did not know how many calories an individual could consume on a daily basis. This is perhaps understandable, since many older people grew up in a period of food shortages rather than excess, and 'junk' food in most places in Mirpur was unheard of,

> "I don't know how many calories we have to take, we don't have much knowledge about this" (female, aged 65)

For these and others, it was not important to know precisely how many calories one should consume, or how many calories are present in a particular food; instead, respondents measured such things according to portions. For example, a 'couple' of samosas or kebabs are fine as a starter followed by a main dish, and this still applies to many Pakistanis, both young and old. Further, foods are cooked according to 'taste', and levels of salt vary considerably between Pakistani families. One observation is that the consumption of salt is higher in Pakistan than Pakistani families in the UK. In Pakistan, a salt plate is always to be found next to a curry. Although I have refrained from 'adding' more salt to a curry, many of my relatives in Pakistan will liberally add more salt to a dish.

In the early days of Pakistani immigration to the UK, it was normal (like in Pakistan) to add extra salt to a dish and this would be on top of curries that already had a fair amount of salt. Although most did not know the amount of salt that was within the healthy range, the younger people did realise they were 'salty'. Letting parents and older people know that a curry had too much salt was pretty much futile. However, during the 1980s onwards, the number of relatives that began to suffer from high blood pressure and diabetes because of a 'bad' diet began a shift in attitudes, particularly mothers and wives who were mainly responsible for cooking.

A husband who had to lower his salt intake on the advice of a doctor struck home the fact that cooking habits had to change and change quickly; for the vast majority of families, they made these changes overnight. The sharing of health information around salt intake quickly spread to friends, family and kinsfolk who accordingly 'lowered' the amount of salt intake. Family discussions around salt intake began to take place openly and it became 'acceptable' to say to someone that their curries had too much salt. It was the genuine desire to 'look after one another' that led to a whole change of cooking habits amongst the Pakistanis. The variation in adding salt, sugar and fats according to taste is important for some,

> "I do not know how many calories we have to use per day. We use salt, sugar and fats according to our taste, some people like more and some less" (male, aged 65)

Similarly, another respondent echoed,

> "I do not know how many calories I need in a day. I don't know how much salt, sugar and fat we need per day, we use them according to our taste and only guess about it" (female, aged 60)

Strong health messages, television documentaries and radio health programmes, particularly those in a community language, are having a positive effect on cooking practices. This has had a particular impact on limiting salt, sugar and fat intake by the majority of Pakistanis. It is interesting to point out that, although many older participants did not speak English, health messages were being translated by siblings, family and friends. In particular, daughters and sons were playing a dominant role in explaining to parents and relatives the importance of reducing key ingredients, in particular salt.

Another major change occurred in the UK, where Pakistani families made a shift from using vegetable ghee to vegetable oil (the latter costs around £7 for a 5-litre bottle) and, for those who can afford it, olive oil. Vegetable ghee has become quite scarce in terms of availability since the majority of Pakistani families have stopped using it. The reason for the sharp decline was as a result of health messages put across to the Pakistani community.

In Pakistan, most families use sunflower oil, which costs around 1200 rupees for a 7-litre container, whereas vegetable ghee costs around 1600 for a 5-kilo container. The transfer of health information from the UK to Pakistan was swift. A sharp increase in sales led to a reduction in the price of vegetable oil, especially in Pakistan, thus becoming within the means of many ordinary Pakistanis. Again, most families cook according to 'taste'; typically, the amount of vegetable ghee used in meat or vegetable dishes was about 200 grams of ghee for each curry. With a litre of vegetable oil, one can normally cook about five dishes.

Reducing sugar and fat in cooking was highlighted by a number of respondents,

> "To some extent I know how many calories we have to use, but we really do not have much knowledge about calories, but I use less sugar and fat" (male, aged 65)

However, one exception to the general consensus was a male respondent, who pointed out that calorie intake depended upon one's gender. Interestingly, he also believed that a young person needs more calories than someone who is older,

> "It depends upon your age and gender, it means a young person needs more calories as compared to someone who is old. A man needs more calories as compared to a woman" (male, aged 60)

This is an illustration of how health messages are being understood by ordinary Pakistanis. One important way of getting the message across to communities is through community centres. In the UK, there are many centres which cater for locals and offer a wide variety of services, for example providing help to claim benefits, or helping people to find a job or a suitable training course. Also, many of them run classes to help the local neighbourhood and the community, for example English lessons, sewing and gym lessons. Thus, community centres act as a place of congregation and a 'meeting place' for locals to come and join in. An abundance of information is shared, from local gossip to important information regarding keeping oneself healthy. Much of this is shared over a cup of tea or whilst learning a new skill. This is particularly useful since the people sharing the information are often knowledgeable about a particular condition, for example diabetes, and they often share information such as causes, symptoms, treatment and long-term effects, particularly if one fails to look after one's diet.

Preference for organic (desi) food

Pakistanis have always had a preference for desi (organic foods), food that is fresh and locally produced. Many families from the 1950s onwards who had a small plot of spare land would cultivate and grow food. The popular foods which they grew included chillies and other vegetables such as potatoes, tomatoes, okra and aubergines. Popular fruits grown in the garden were apples, oranges, satsumas and pears. All of these are seasonal fruits and vegetables and require little maintenance. The following respondent is typical of most Pakistanis when she makes a link between being 'healthy' and food being 'fresh'.

> "I think the food we are eating is healthy because we eat fresh food" (female, aged 65)

Again, food that is 'fresh' and had 'taste' was preferred,

> "We enjoy eating only simple desi (organic) food because it's fresh and also very tasty" (female, aged 65)

Another respondent echoes the importance of purchasing a variety of foods. It is the variety of foods that the family is able to afford that still largely determines a person's wealth, as the following quotes show,

> "I enjoy eating all types of food, but I like the meat more as compared to other types of foods" (male, aged 65)

> "Like meat, vegetables, pulses and beans and sometimes sweets" (female, aged 61)

Similarly,

> "Mostly I like to eat meat and fruits" (male, aged 65)

Also important was being in a financial position to be able to eat organically, especially food that is grown on one's land,

> "I buy the organic food, we buy all types of organic food like meat, eggs poultry and vegetables. Fifty per cent of the food we buy is organic and fifty per cent we produce our own" (male, aged 65)

Keeping chickens at home is another symbol of wealth among families in Pakistan, as is being able to consume fresh eggs on a daily basis,

> "We buy organic food because at home we have less quantities of food to fulfil our needs. We buy all types of organic food like chicken, eggs and vegetables" (male, aged 65)

In light of the upheaval of families moving to larger towns and cities in search of work and better opportunities, some of the early preferences of growing food at home have largely all but disappeared. This does not mean that eating organically produced foods has given way to mass-produced markets and preferences. The following respondent highlights that, when he cannot produce enough organic foods, he compensates this by purchasing extra food at the local market,

> "We buy all types of organic foods like meat, vegetables and fruits except eggs and chicken. Mostly we grow our own organic food but it is not enough to fulfil our needs, so we have to buy vegetables, fruits and meat" (male, aged 63)

> "We have to buy from outside because I cannot produce enough to sustain myself. I like to eat desi food so this encourages me to buy it" (female, aged 62)

The next respondent reveals an indication of change over generations,

> "We don't depend on ourselves to produce the food so we buy more from outside" (female, aged 62)

Another female respondent expressed the preference to produce as much as they can on their own land,

> "We have organic food at our home, we have cultivated vegetables in our small garden and we have hens at home so that we don't have to buy eggs from the shops" (female, aged 65)

This respondent lived in one of the smaller villages on the outskirts of Mirpur, having lived in the same village for 60 years. Being resourceful was a skill that most Pakistani families learnt, especially during the years after Independence in 1947. Food was at a premium and the ability to grow some fruit and vegetables in their gardens was a golden opportunity that only a few families could afford to miss. Those who could afford to keep hens at home had the opportunity to eat meat every so often.

However, there are signs of change so, although the young prefer desi (organic) foods, there is some reluctance to grow them at home; instead, they want to purchase them from a local producer. This is perhaps understandable given that the young will be doing some form of paid work and either have little time to cultivate fruit and vegetables at home, or simply do not have the energy to do so after a long, hard day. The older generation who were interviewed for this research will continue to do so for as long as their health is good. Some, however, were fortunate enough to be able to employ someone to help grow and manage the land.

Eating desi (organic) foods

Most participants said they eat 'mostly' organic foods because of the benefits to one's health, thus encouraging a family to buy more. Respondents did not like chemicals sprayed onto fruit and vegetables to help them grow. Chemicals are seen as being detrimental to one's health and to be avoided as much as possible. Older Pakistanis were raised on desi food and they always have believed that it gave them strength to do a day's hard work. This still holds true for most older Pakistanis,

> "Mostly we eat organic food because it is good for your health so it encourages me to buy more" (male, aged 65)

Most believe that a Western diet contains too many chemicals and harmful ingredients and has led to conditions such as diabetes.

> "Now people like to buy more than earlier because they have more money and the taste of the food has changed as well because of the chemicals in the food" (female, aged 62)

The young people in Pakistan (and those who can afford it) see fast foods which are high in salt, sugar and fat as being everyday foods, readily accessible and available 24/7.

Types of foods consumed

Exploring the issue of what older Pakistanis enjoy eating revealed interesting insights into their eating habits. Some habits still hold true for many respondents, for example when they mentioned they do not like to eat 'sweets or drink sweet drinks'. This cut across all socio backgrounds and gender,

> "I do not like to eat (Pakistani) sweets or drink sweet drinks or any other food" (male, aged 65)

For others, eating 'simple foods' is still important, as is avoiding fizzy drinks and (Pakistani) sweets, which are very high in sugar and fat content,

> "We like to eat simple foods and very rarely we have fizzy drinks and (Pakistani) sweets, they are only for the children" (female, aged 60)

For others it was much more infrequent, perhaps once a week or once every fortnight,

> "We rarely eat sweets and have drinks maybe once in a week or after two weeks" (female, aged 65)

Sweets (Pakistani) are eaten on a regular basis and particularly during celebrations, such as births and marriages. For those relatives and friends attending a celebration it is customary to bring a box of Pakistani sweets, usually a mixture of hard and soft sweets. Those with a 'really sweet tooth' are attracted to these sweets because of their very high sugar and fat content. However, for some they are one of the 'forbidden' foods and because they see the need to control their diet and well-being. However, some older people have continued to enjoy a variety of such foods over the years and because of their continued good health,

> "We eat all types of foods like drinks, sweets and all other types of foods that are available in the market" (female, aged 61)

Health messages that encourage older Pakistanis to reduce high sugar and fat content foods have had a limited effect on some. This is not because of the lack of trying on the part of the individual, or family members not helping, but the need for one-to-one professional help over a period of weeks and months.

What food would you like to eat?

Those families with a good income were able to purchase whatever they liked, most preferring meat over a vegetable curry. For these respondents, a meat or chicken curry contained little 'water' or vegetables such as potatoes,

> "I enjoy eating meat and money is not affecting my buying power and I like to eat vegetables as well, but I like meat more" (male, aged 65)

Similarly,

> "I enjoy eating all kinds of foods. I eat what I want and whatever is good for my health, at this stage money is not a factor" (male, aged 60)

However, those families who could rarely afford to have a meat curry often put in vegetables such as cauliflower or potatoes to make the curry last. For a family of six people, each person would get about two pieces of chicken or meat and a few potatoes,

> "The foods I would like to eat but cannot afford to eat so money is a factor which affects what we buy" (male, aged 63)

Pakistan does not have a system of credit and everything has to be paid for 'in cash and on the spot'. However, those with a local families with good social status in the community are allowed to purchase on 'tick', settling their account every few weeks. Overseas Pakistanis are nearly always allowed to purchase on 'tick', some settling their account at the end of their stay in Pakistan. Many years ago, all families bought household goods on credit and repaid as and when they were able to do. This is an illustration of kin members helping each other during times of financial hardship. The essential goods such a flour, sugar, salt, butter and oil are always on credit.

In reality, many families had to compromise in order to stay within their monthly budget and what they could afford. Diet for poorer families was changeable month by month depending on their fortunes the previous month. It was important for families not to overstretch their spending power and to put some money aside in case it was needed, for example in case of urgent medical treatment for a family member,

> "Sometimes the food I enjoy eating we cannot afford to do, so we have to compromise to whatever is affordable" (male, aged 63)

In Pakistan, one does not have a mortgage since the individual buys the land in cash and then builds a house, again in cash; also, there is no council tax to pay. In reality, and especially for poorer families, they pay for the important things first, which include: rent, water to be delivered to their home, a gas cylinder to cook food. Other essential bills that may need to be paid are: medical bills, doctors and school fees. After paying for these essentials, then the family buys food, carefully working out their affordability on a daily or weekly basis. Spending power varied enormously for most Mirpuris, as few have long-term employment contracts, for example those employed in the local government and banks. As discussed above, for the rest of the population work is dependent wholly on daily or weekly contractual work and local conditions vary.

Consuming fruit

Fruit is available in abundance in Pakistan because of its hot climate. As discussed above, most respondents prefer to eat desi (organic) fruit while others grow fruit on their own land. Limes and lemons are very popular in the hot summers, where it is not uncommon for temperatures to reach 40 degrees Celsius; most Pakistanis make lemonade with crushed ice to cool themselves and is a great alternative to drinking fizzy drinks. Others prefer the following in the summer months,

> "I eat oranges, grapes and pomegranates and apples as well, also watermelon and melons" (male, aged 65)

Pakistanis eat fruits according to the season. The following respondent also mentioned eating fruit that is grown on their land,

> "I eat apples, bananas and all seasonal fruits like mangoes, grapes, watermelon and plums. We eat some quantity of fruits that is available at home" (female, aged 60)

Similarly, another respondent said,

> "I eat fruit mostly, I like to eat good quality of apples, pomegranate and all other seasonal fruits like organic and mangoes. I eat fruit every day" (male, aged 65)

For the following respondent, eating fruit that was in season was important, as were the health benefits,

> "I eat all types of fruits like apples, oranges, grapes and mangoes and all types of seasonal foods. I like fruits because it is good for my health" (male, aged 60)

Much of the solid food in Mirpur is supplied by a number local farmers; in fact, it is common for local farmers to supply fresh fruit and vegetables to local towns and villages across Pakistan. In this way, locals are assured of the quality of the food they are purchasing.

Eating Five-a-Day

The cost of food has risen globally and this has had an enormous knock-on effect on most families in Mirpur. Eating fruit on a daily basis is becoming a struggle for an increasing number of people. For example, a kilo of apples and pears costs 1200 rupees (approx.), a dozen bananas or oranges cost 1500 rupees (approx.), a kilo of guavas 1000 rupees and a kilo of grapes around 800 rupees. A watermelon costs 100-150 rupees and a honeydew melon costs 200 rupees. The most expensive fruit are mangoes, a kilo of which costs around 2,000 rupees. Given the 'high' prices of fruit, most Pakistanis are unable to afford to eat anywhere near five-a-day – unless, of course, as discussed above, one is able to grow fruit on their own land. In terms of consuming fruit, the picture was varied; there were participants who had a choice of eating whatever they liked and ate as frequently as they wished,

> "I eat five-a-day whatever I like every day, I eat it but sometimes I give it a miss" (female, aged 60)

Similarly,

> "Sometimes I can eat five-a-day" (female, aged 61)

It was common for some participants (and family members) to have fruit either during breakfast or later in the morning. Many had an orange or a couple of small bananas before they set off to work in the morning,

> "I eat fruits daily maybe twice or once a day like in the morning and in the evening as well" (ibid)

When visitors arrive, it is common for the host to serve fruit to their guests; these usually comprise oranges and apples and, on a hot day, it is common to serve a watermelon which would have been left in the fridge. Fruit was eaten at different times of the day, depending upon one's need and also other factors, such as the weather,

> "I do not eat five-a-day. I eat two fruits a day like in the morning and in the evenings" (male, aged 65)

However, a number of older respondents ate fruit during the morning or in the evening,

> "As a routine I eat them along with my meal or during the morning time sometimes at night" (female, aged 62)

While others ate fewer than five-a-day,

> "I do not eat five-a-day. I eat twice or sometimes three in a day" (male, aged 65)

Fruit was bought on a regular basis. Some bought it daily, while others twice weekly, as the following female respondent revealed,

> "I buy the fruit twice a week and enjoy eating apples and bananas; usually it's one portion a day or sometimes more" (female, aged 65)

Shopping daily had its advantages. For one thing, they purchased only the freshest of fruits; however, and especially for older participants, it meant that, by walking to the bazaar, it enabled them to exercise for a period of time. Also, it allowed them to socialise with friends and family; especially in Pakistan, it would be unusual not to meet anyone you knew whilst going out to shop in a locality where 'everyone knows everyone'. In fact, shopping is a key area where people meet and discuss everything from the price of fruit to the price of gas! It is a social space to meet people; for others, they sit outside the café enjoying a cup of Asian-style tea and watch the world go by. Among the participants, there were many others who struggled financially to eat any fruit, or it was irregular,

> "I eat fruits, I eat apples, oranges and fruits which are affordable for me. I eat fruit once a week or every two weeks and sometimes may be every weeks it is not regular" (male, aged 63)

Consuming meat

There is a 'hierarchy' of curry dishes. The least expensive dish to cook is a very simple yoghurt curry with a few spices costing around 30 rupees, followed by potato and spinach curry (100 rupees), potato and peas curry (120 rupees), followed by lentil curries (different variations) costing around 120 rupees; a chicken costs about 1500 rupees and meat can easily cost 1500 rupees a kilo. The local shops are usually slightly cheaper than those based in the shopping marts. It is not unsurprising that only the most affluent are able to consume chicken and meat curries on a regular basis.

Without question, the vast majority of Pakistanis, if given the choice, would prefer a meat dish. The following respondent, given his financial position, could afford meat every day,

> "I like to eat desi (organic) chicken, mutton and beef. I eat meat regularly like twice or even three times in a day" (male, aged 60)

Another respondent said,

> "I like to eat meat probably too much. I eat all types of meat but mostly I like cow meat. I eat it twice or three times a week and I eat chicken as well" (male, aged 65)

In my personal experience, I have never come across an individual who was a vegetarian or a vegan. For most, they would eat meat every day if finances allowed. There was some variation in types of meat consumed,

> "I eat meat and I like cow and buffalo meat" (male, aged 65)

While others also preferred delicacies such as goat meat,

> "I enjoy eating chicken and meat like goat, buffalo and bull meat. I eat mostly chicken meat once a week sometimes twice a week" (female, aged 65)

Affordability is a major factor. A typical family of six people would need around two kilos of meat, which would last them a day at the most,

> "I eat meat, I eat beef, mutton and chicken. We eat meat every two weeks or maybe every four weeks, it depends upon our buying power and when it is affordable" (male, aged 63)

In Pakistan, families have roti and curry twice a day and they eat until they are completely full, thus for most there is little need to have snacks throughout the day. Most Mirpuri families will cook enough to last for one meal, for example lunch. The evening meal will again be cooked fresh. This is especially applicable to day labourers who work away from home; they usually take their lunch with them, for example a curry dish, several rotis and something sweet, if available, in their tin pots.

The preference for most Pakistanis is 'home' cooked food and this is definitely over fast food or restaurant food, which some consider as being inferior in quality and nutrients. Also, it is cheaper than buying food at the fast food outlet; if they give into temptation whilst working away, they will usually have a portion of samosas and pakoras because they are filling and will usually get them through the long, hot summer's day in Mirpur. However, fruits such as a couple of slices of ice-cooled watermelon are commonly purchased. As regards drinks, the most favoured is plain cold water, which is relatively cheap to purchase followed by the different variations of fizzy drinks.

Consuming vegetables

As discussed above, most Pakistanis prefer a chicken or meat dish over a vegetable curry. Vegetable curries are usually cooked in addition to a meat curry, almost like a side dish for those who want to taste something different. For example, a typical man in Pakistan can consume three rotis;

he will usually have two roti with a meat dish and one or a half a roti with a vegetable curry. Again, it is important to remember that, the more affluent the family, the more dishes are prepared; secondly, only a small number of families are in this position.

In the UK, whilst visiting relatives, it would not be uncommon to see the following foods laid out on the table: a chicken or meat dish, a vegetable curry, a lentil curry, pilau rice with chicken or meat, samosas, sweet rice, pakoras and fizzy drinks. Although salad is usually also served, it is normally the last to be consumed.

Like the cost of chicken and meat, the price of vegetables has also increased quite considerably over the last few years. In Pakistan, the following are the prices for essential vegetables used for making a curry. The prices are in rupees for a kilo: cauliflower 50 rupees; potatoes 35 rupees; onions 35 rupees; tomatoes 100 rupees; green chillies 40 rupees; garlic 300 rupees; aubergines 200 rupees and okra 450 rupees. Vegetable dishes are served in addition to meat dishes; favourite dishes are spinach and cauliflower dishes, both with potato,

> "We eat vegetables and we use it along with meat as well" (female, aged 60)

Some respondents preferred a vegetable curry as much as a meat dish,

> "I eat all types of vegetables which are available, mostly I like to eat spinach and cauliflower. I eat vegetables twice or three times a week" (male, aged 65)

Variation in terms of dishes prepared was important for most respondents given that they have two different curries a day. The usual practice would be to have a vegetable curry for lunch and then a chicken or meat dish in the evening,

> "I eat vegetables in our home. We eat all types of vegetables like spinach, peas, potatoes and cauliflower. We eat vegetables twice a week with rice and whichever fresh vegetables are available in the market" (male, aged 65)

'Variation' was important for older people (if they had the financial resources) given that most of them did not eat fast foods. Mixing vegetable and meat dishes at regular intervals meant that they still held some excitement for the next meal,

> "I enjoy eating vegetables. I like them better now than before. I like to eat peas, potatoes, pumpkins and spinach. I eat them about three time or twice in a week" (male, aged 60)

Again,

> "We eat okra, spinach, potatoes, cauliflower and cabbage. We eat it twice or three times in a week" (female, aged 60)

The young people did enjoy a variation, albeit replacing 'healthier' home-cooked foods with a takeaway. Typically, and those who had the financial resources, they would have fast foods several times a week.

Consuming lentils

The least expensive of all the dishes are lentils (includes all varieties). They are also the cheapest dish to prepare, requiring the very basic of ingredients such as onions, garlic, coriander and salt and pepper. Some families, because of cost and who need to make the curry last, will add water.

The quality of lentils varies enormously depending upon the resources of the family. In Pakistan, one can purchase two differing qualities of lentils. The 'number one' is a genuine variety; it has been processed, cleaned and washed and produced to a high quality. The 'number two', however, is of a much lower quality and it is not uncommon for these lentils to contain dirt and stones; therefore it is reflected in the price.

Lentils are really useful, as are kidney beans; they can be prepared as a lentil curry with roti, or often with boiled rice and served with a simple salad including onions, tomatoes and lettuce and perhaps also a 'watery' mint sauce. If available, the family will replace water with sweet yoghurt, again ensuring 'taste',

> "We eat lentils and pulses and beans, we only eat two or three types of pulses. We eat them once a week sometimes along with rice" (male, aged 65)

Again, another respondent echoed a similar diet,

> "We eat all types of lentils, beans and pulses and we eat it twice or three times a week. Families like us depend on lentils and pulses" (male, aged 63)

Much rarer was the practice of mixing lentils with vegetables or meat. This was done to 'bulk' up the curry so it was something like a stew, especially when water was added,

> "Usually we eat it once a week so it's regular and sometimes we mix it with vegetables" (ibid)

For many, lentils were consumed infrequently, especially among families who had a reasonable income,

> "Very rarely I eat lentils, pulses and beans. Sometimes I eat them every two weeks or once in a week" (male, aged 65)

Similarly,

> "I do not eat lentils, pulses or beans, sometimes I eat beans but very rarely" (male, aged 60)

Changes in diet over time

It was interesting to note the generational change. The older generation, which made up most of the the respondents in this research, grew up in a time of enormous uncertainty. Respondents in their mid-60s were born just after Independence (1947) when Pakistan was created. There was uncertainty over where families would settle in the newly-formed country and food was largely scarce except for the most affluent of families. In the early years after Independence, one's 'diet' comprised of very basic foods.

Many respondents had noticed the change over time. A regular income ensures the family can have stability, thus pay for essential bills and food. The concern for many Pakistani families is that their diet changes very frequently, perhaps daily or on a weekly basis, depending upon how much the family can set aside for food. Buying power is essential, as the following respondent points out,

> "I think my diet has changed over time. It is because now we depend more on our buying power and the young people do not like to eat desi foods so diet has changed" (male, aged 65)

He also mentions the preference of older Pakistanis for desi (organic) foods, but the younger people have developed a taste for different foods. This is not to say the young have completely disowned desi foods, but they have incorporated other types of foods such as fast food and a Western dict,

> "My diet has changed over time, the diet has changed due to two reasons. First we mostly depend on our buying power and secondly we do not produce our own food" (male, aged 63)

As discussed above, fewer Pakistani families grow their own food except for the basics such as mint, coriander and tomatoes. Time is an important factor where the young perhaps have less time to look after the garden or a smallholding like their parents. Also, financial income is important as those who can afford to buy from the shops do so; it is a sign of affordability.

Another respondent explains changes in eating habits over time from eating 'simple foods', perhaps a roti and mint sauce, to present times where people can afford to diversify their diet. Trying different foods, especially Western foods, is a sign of affordability and affiliation. It is not uncommon for a Pakistani family to go out to a restaurant for pasta and pizza dressed in Western clothes (especially the father and children); until recently, this would have been unheard of. Consuming Western foods encapsulate all things that most young people desire,

> "My diet has changed over time because in the past people ate simple foods, but now people can afford to eat differently. Nowadays we eat takeaway food such as sweets and the second reason we use chemicals" (male, aged 60)

As mentioned above, consuming 'Western foods' such as fish and chips and pizza represents a change from a diet of traditional foods and also represents affluence, because such foods are expensive compared to 'Asian' foods. In fact, for many Pakistanis purchasing Western foods is beyond their means. The desire to consume such foods is clear.

Dietary change over time

A change in dietary habits over time was particularly noted by most of the Mirpuri respondents; this had become more prevalent as they saw a change in the food tastes of the younger generation. Equally, they also saw a change in how food was grown, as the demand to feed an increasing population has led to the use of chemicals being used to aid growth of fruit and vegetables. This was considered a change for the worse for many respondents,

> "I think the diet has changed from being better to worse because of the chemicals we have started using in our foods" (male, aged 65)

Similarly, another remarks a change for the worse from eating 'pure' foods to using 'chemicals',

> "The diet has changed from it being better to worse because we use chemicals. In the past we ate pure (desi) food and now we cannot eat pure food" (male, aged 63)

For the following respondent, it was not only the chemicals that were used on crops but the fast pace of life was highlighted. Again, as the above respondents discussed, all this was considered a change for the worse,

> "It is because of the fast pace of life now people have less time to produce their own food or they want their food quickly so they use more chemicals; this is one way you can say my diet has changed from better to worse" (male, aged 65)

Again,

> "People should eat desi food and try to eat fresh food this way it would be healthier for them" (female, aged 65)

For the above respondent, she associated desi foods with being healthy. It was not the fact that older people were turning away from fast foods and takeaways, but the preparation of food. The demand for fresh foods is considerable and many Pakistanis, irrespective of income, are still willing to pay more for desi foods.

How do you think people can be encouraged to eat healthily?

One of the most important health challenges facing governments across the world is to encourage individuals to eat healthily. The pressure of leading a busy life was an important variable that meant some people ignored living a healthy lifestyle. However, it is also about educating the population about healthy living. The following respondent points out the need to educate people about leading a healthy lifestyle. Considering what one eats and engaging in some form of physical activity should both be complementary,

> "We are too busy in our daily activities and we do not think about our health; there is a need to educate people" (male, aged 60)

For others, it was simply being 'lazy', which led to some individuals failing to change their dietary habits,

> "If people think about their health they should be encouraged to eat healthily. It is our laziness and our tastes that have changed and people mostly do not think about their health" (male, aged 65)

The above male respondent mentions "tastes have changed", suggesting a shift from eating fresh, healthier foods to consuming takeaways or fast foods. Similarly, some respondents suggested the strong need to receive education about diet and physical activity,

> "Perhaps if we individually go to people or there should be special teams telling them about what they should eat. In this way people could be encouraged to eat healthily" (male, aged 65)

The most favoured method of receiving health information was face to face communication. This was echoed by many respondents irrespective of their literacy levels or socioeconomic background,

> "Like you have come to me for the interview likewise there should be teams to make people aware to educate the people, so in this way people can be encouraged to eat healthily" (male, aged 63)

The hope for respondents was that it would make the population aware of the dangers of leading an unhealthy lifestyle and the likelihood of getting diseases such as diabetes and heart disease,

> "If we made people aware about the spread of certain diseases" (male, aged 62)

Equally, although some of the methods of reaching out to communities were obvious, the difficult task was 'reaching out' to the population in a way that would lead them to making a positive change. This is about proactive engagement with communities who live in remote regions of Pakistan and have little access to health services. Despite the effort of health agencies, some felt they are constantly competing against the odds,

> "People can be encouraged if they took note of their health, but nowadays people do not think about their health so it's hard to encourage them" (female, aged 61)

Making changes to one's dietary habits requires change on a micro level, a community by community approach. It requires a focussed approach with all members of each community getting involved, including elders, community leaders, grandparents, parents and young people. Further, and crucially, parents play an enormous part in what their families eat, as they do the shopping and the cooking. Even slight modifications can have a major impact on one's health, for example a reduction in salt and sugar.

CHAPTER SEVEN

PHYSICAL ACTIVITY

> "Exercise is most important for one's health so everyone should exercise, especially if they are becoming overweight" (female, aged 62)

Cultural factors: Early experiences of Pakistani women (Din, 2006)

Culturally, norms and attitudes have largely dictated the practices of the biraderi (kin) and the community. Females have been largely prevented from going outside of the compounds of the house for all but essential visits, for example a visit to the doctor or the dentist. Going out of the house to engage in physical activity is rare except amongst the higher socioeconomic groups.

The following is a section from Din (2006) describing the early experiences of Pakistani women. The early experience of Pakistani women was one of isolation. The Pakistani women, who arrived in the UK, experienced extreme loneliness and were unable to leave the house without their husbands. Pakistani women were not only restricted by the practice of purdah, but also by their lack of English skills (Rose et al., 1969).

Khan (1979) found that, on the arrival of Pakistani women into Britain, they reinforced the Muslim culture, where they were kept in strict purdah and were isolated from the local indigenous population (Din, 2006). The arrival of immigrant women and children meant the strict segregation of activities between males and females within the Pakistani household and that male members worked and spent their leisure in the company of other men (Allen, 1971). However, there are strong signs of cultural change: the experiences of rural women differ from those of a middle-class background, where many women from prosperous backgrounds, for example from Islamabad and Karachi, are working or attending university and participating in leisure activities. There are complex inheritances that remain significant in the present day and the consequences can still be seen (Din, 2006).

Do you think you are healthy?

There was an in-depth discussion with respondents around the state of the health of participants. A number of participants felt that their health was less than good and certainly compared to when they were younger and youthful,

> "I am not healthy I have a heart problem and urine problem as well" (male, aged 62)

Similarly,

> "I have problems like breathing difficulties and blood pressure" (female, aged 62)

Others thought they were 'healthy' apart from occasional headaches. The concern here was the male respondent who suffered from blood pressure, but otherwise feels healthy,

> "I think I am healthy but sometimes I suffer from headaches or blood pressure, otherwise I am healthy" (male, aged 63)

The struggle on the part of respondents to attempt to engage in some form of physical activity, despite having medical conditions, was evident,

> "I have some conditions including blood pressure and heart problems. I do not exercise, I only walk, but I cannot go far and sometimes I do the housework" (female, aged 61)

Others attempted to avoid foods that were considered to be unsuitable because of their health condition,

> "I take care of my health and try to avoid such foods and are not suitable for me because I have problems with blood pressure" (male, aged 60)

It is interesting to note with the above two examples that respondents were being proactive, whether engaging in some physical activity or dietary changes that would alleviate the symptoms. Respondents were in a position to offer family members and friends advice about making wrong health choices, especially a sedentary lifestyle. There were a small number of respondents that led an active lifestyle, one which incorporated a healthy diet coupled with physical activity,

> "I think I feel healthy because I take care of myself" (male, aged 65)

Physical activity

Among the respondents who said they exercised, they engaged in a number of different exercises whether this was using an exercise bike, going for a walk in the park or doing the housework and was done on a regular basis.

The following respondent had a lifetime routine of regular exercising, often on a daily basis, and he was the only respondent who did weight training and push ups,

> "I regularly exercise, I exercise in my home I have exercise equipment I walk daily as well and at home I do weight-training" (male, aged 60)

While another respondent was thinking of purchasing exercise equipment,

> "I exercise regularly so this encourages me to do more. I am thinking of buying fitness tools so then I will be able to exercise more easily and this will make it easier for me" (male, aged 65)

A common activity among the majority of male respondents was going to the park for a walk. However, for many this was a stroll in the park rather than a brisk walk. Walking is a communal activity in Pakistan, especially after the main evening meal. Most say it helps one to digest the evening meal. This is especially popular in the summer months, when temperatures often reach 40 degrees Celsius in the afternoon and 25 Celsius in the evening,

> "I exercise regularly. I exercise at home or sometimes I go to the park" (male, aged 65)

Similarly,

> "The only exercise I do is that I walk daily" (female, aged 62)

While others used the opportunity to walk to the mosque for daily prayers,

> "I do not exercise regularly, however I try to walk where I have to go outside like when I go to the mosque daily" (male, aged 62)

Similarly, although the following respondent did not go to a gym to exercise, he walked daily in addition to getting some exercise whilst doing the housework. 'Housework' is a flexible term which incorporates all types of housework including cleaning, washing-up but also attending to one's garden and land. The following respondent owned a large plot attached to the house on which he kept cows, sheep and goats, while another section of the land was used for growing fruit and vegetables. In this case, he had oranges, lemons and lime trees, and lettuce, cauliflower, okra and aubergines in the far corner of his plot. Attending to the vegetation allowed him to have enough exercise,

> "No, I do not exercise. I do not go anywhere for exercise. I do walk daily so I do this type of exercise and do my housework as well" (male, aged 65)

However, for other respondents they simply walked for long distances,

> "I do not exercise, I do not go anyway to exercise and there is no trend for exercising here. I only walk where I have to; daily I walk about one mile or sometimes maybe more so I do this type of exercise" (male, aged 63)

Others highlighted that going to the gym to exercise was not a trend in their village. This was something echoed especially by older female respondents. Cultural attitudes largely prevented females from going outside of the house to exercise; unfortunately, these cultural norms and attitudes are still prevalent in some villages and towns across Pakistan,

> "I worry about not exercising but I cannot exercise. I would not like to go to any fitness centre to exercise, it's not the trend here especially someone at my age" (female, aged 61)

Frequency of physical activity

For the male respondents, strenuous physical activity was mainly done through working as a day labourer typically working 12 to 14 hours a day. There is no retirement age in Pakistan (except for those in civil service and the financial sector, normally retiring after 25 years of service). For most, they continue to work until their health suffers or if they have son(s) who is/are able to support the family. The following respondent continued his exercise regime from working as a day labourer to engaging in physical activity,

> "I have been exercising regularly for the past fifteen years and before I did not exercise regularly, however at that time I had done hard work and it was good for me" (male, aged 60)

Similarly,

> "I have never exercised regularly during my life but I have done hard work during my life and I have lifted heavy goods" (male, aged 65)

'Health' status was often linked to the job performed by the respondent before retiring, as the following respondent explains. Being in the army ensured that he continued to lead a physically active lifestyle,

> "I was in the army so I regularly exercised till now, so this is the reason for my fitness" (male, aged 65)

While many females used the opportunity to exercise by running an often very busy household, which ensured they were keeping active through doing daily household chores,

> "I do not exercise, I only do the housework regularly this is the exercise I do" (female, aged 65)

Do you worry about not exercising?

It was interesting to note that few respondents said they worried about not exercising and believed that going for a stroll to the park, mosque or to the bazaar provided all the physical exercise they needed. Much of this was leisurely walking rather than brisk walking,

> "I do not worry about not exercising because I walk a lot so it is enough for me" (male, aged 65)

Again,

> "I regularly exercise so I do not worry" (male, aged 65)

Many of the respondents had gained weight especially when they reached their 50s. Some had given up work because of ill health, while others were working reduced hours or working during the colder autumn and winter months rather than working under the blistering hot summers of Pakistan. Others and those who were fortunate enough to retire took the opportunity gladly. For this group, this was followed by a sedentary lifestyle, having little to do during the day except socialising with friends and family. What is clear is that the motivations to exercise were different, depending upon socioeconomic circumstances and gender of participants.

Going to a gym

Further differences were found when respondents were asked whether they attend or have been members of the gym. Engaging in physical activity was seen as something to be done in the privacy of one's home and this was particularly correct in this sample of older respondents, with the exception of ‘walking’, as discussed above.

There are several privately owned ‘gyms’ in Mirpur which predominantly cater for young males, though some have separate facilities for females. All are welcome to attend. Also, there are many college and University gyms which cater for the needs of students. Young people are the main drivers for health changes and also the main medium in which health messages are delivered to parents and older relatives in Pakistan, particularly those who do not read English. Most private schools and all colleges and Universities use English as the medium for teaching. With Internet access especially at educational establishments, young people can learn about health conditions and diseases in a way that their parents could not ever have imagined. Much of this information is shared with biraderi members.

The advantage of the Internet is that information can be accessed 24/7 as opposed to going to a government-run clinic or hospital, which often involves travel and time. Most ‘hits’ are about diabetes, heart disease and cancer with increasing number of Pakistanis been affected; also, the ways in which slight changes in diet or physical activity can go a long way in preventing some conditions. Particularly effective has been limiting salt and vegetable ghee in cooking; most have changed to vegetable oil while others with limited family incomes rely on less expensive ghee to do their cook.

A typical response to the question about whether they go to the gym or not was,

> “I do not go to any fitness centres here and I am not interested to go anywhere” (male, aged 65)

Similarly, another respondent said,

> “I would not want to attend any fitness centre to do any exercises” (male, aged 65)

For some, they used their age to justify not going to the gym. This attitude has been a major cultural barrier for health promotion teams everywhere that going to the gym is for younger people,

> “There is a fitness centre here in Mirpur and mostly the younger generation has now started to attend the fitness centres” (male, aged 60)

This is equally applicable to the situation in the UK, where cultural attitudes deter older people from exercising publicly,

> "I would not like to attend a fitness centre to exercise and mostly the people at my age do not like to go for exercise" (male, aged 63)

Another respondent echoed,

> "I do exercises at home so I would not like to attend a fitness centre" (male, aged 60)

While this response was typical of most female respondents,

> "At my age I wouldn't want to attend any fitness centres" (female, aged 62)

Fitness centres in Mirpur

One of the main problems in Pakistan is information receiving, especially among families where illiteracy is high. By contrast, as discussed earlier, families that have members who can read Urdu and especially English have benefited, whether being able to access information on the Internet or to read about health conditions.

Illiteracy is a major problem in Pakistan, especially in rural villages and towns, and it is not uncommon for generations of the same family not to have had any form of schooling. Until recently, schooling was the privilege of the affluent classes. Typical private school fees vary from anywhere between 5,000 to 15,000 rupees. In addition to paying for the school uniform, textbooks, lunch and transport, costs can quite easily add up to 3,000 rupees on top of the monthly fees. Thus, schooling in Pakistan has been out of reach of the ordinary family who struggle with high unemployment, or those who are in employment with low wages. Wages sometimes barely cover the monthly essentials such as rent, food and utilities.

A number of state schools have been established to try and ensure the new generation of Pakistanis receive some elementary schooling, thus increasing literacy levels, particularly in rural areas. Despite free school provision, families from poorer backgrounds still struggle to send their children to school. However, families still have to pay for the school uniforms and textbooks, which can amount to a hefty monthly sum and is money that can be better spent elsewhere on basic essentials such as food. There is another economic reason.

In households where the mother has learnt a skill such as seamstressing, her older female siblings will look after younger brothers and sisters whilst she works. Older siblings are expected to contribute fully to the running of the household, while cooking and cleaning is shared among the siblings. Every member of the family has a task to do. The older girls will predominately look after the home and the sons will go and do the daily shopping or run errands. To increase the family's income, teenage sons from poorer backgrounds will go along with their father to help. For example, if the father is employed as a decorator, the son can help his dad to prepare the room for painting and help to move furniture so the job will be done quicker. In this case, earning money or helping parents takes precedence over schooling, but one can understand why.

Attending a fitness centre was for the privilege of the few, even when it was in the interest of one's health. The finances simply did not allow one to join,

> "I do not have information about any fitness centres here because I am not interested in going there. I could afford to go to a fitness centre so cost would not be a factor affecting to go there" (male, aged 65)

In the UK, there is a strong push towards physical activity and interventions are designed to help individuals to engage in exercise, and schemes such as Exercise on Prescription have encouraged this. This is in contrast to the situation in Pakistan,

> "Maybe there are fitness centres in Mirpur. I could not afford to attend the fitness centre even if I wanted to" (male, aged 63)

A strong undercurrent of prevalent cultural beliefs continues to play a major part in discouraging healthy behaviours,

> "I don't have any knowledge about any fitness clubs I don't have any reason to be" (female, aged 65)

For some, although finances allowed them to attend a gym, they did not take the opportunity,

> "There are fitness centres in Mirpur. I can afford to go to the fitness centre and money does not affect my decision" (male, aged 65)

Respondents realised the benefits of engaging in some form of physical activity, whether it was going to the gym, working out at home or doing gardening. For those who are suffering from conditions such as type 2 diabetes, they accepted the health messages and were trying to change habits of a lifetime and proactively engaging in exercising. Advice from health professionals was, in some cases, beginning to be accepted,

> "My doctor told me about the importance of doing exercises and the effect it can have on my health" (male, aged 60)

Similarly,

> "I know the importance of exercise so this encourages me to exercise so I walk every day. It is easy for me to walk so this is the easiest way" (male, aged 63)

Coupled with dietary changes, they hoped it would bring about good health and hopefully a regime that is sustainable. Good health meant being able to support one's family and being able to engage in family and community events. Good health also meant fewer visits to the doctor and the health clinic, particularly important in Pakistan where visits to the doctor have to be paid for. Medical bills for conditions such as type 1 diabetes, where insulin has to be paid for, run into thousands of rupees a month. This is often beyond the reach of most Pakistani families.

Increasing the level of physical activity

Encouraging people to engage in physical activity has become a global goal, especially in the Western world, which has seen a considerable rise in obesity. Physical activity coupled with limited dietary controls is seen as a global target. Getting numerous health messages across to populations is straightforward. However, changing behaviours and attitudes amongst individuals and groups is much more difficult, especially in marginalised and excluded communities. Interventions that look into ways of physical activity appear to achieve results; however, once the intervention or the study stops, individuals are left struggling. Interventional studies can offer new possibilities to those taking part; for some it's a great motivator, while for others they offer hope. What achieves goals is sustainability in the long run.

While having discussions with participants about ways of encouraging healthy behaviours, it led to a discussion of cultural beliefs. There was a clear gender divide. The male respondents believed that there are no cultural barriers that prevent individuals from participating in recreational activities, irrespective of one's gender. However, the female respondents were of the opposite opinion, in that cultural norms and attitudes dictate what is acceptable or not.

The following male respondent remarks on the importance of doing 'hard work', in this case manual labour, and if one was unemployed then they should try and exercise by way of walking,

> "People should do hard work if they are not exercising and if we encourage them to do more walking in this way people can be encouraged to participate in it" (male, aged 65)

He continued by saying that there are no cultural barriers that restrict individuals from engaging in exercise,

> "There is no cultural barrier, everyone is free to do exercise, there is no restriction in our religion for exercising but our religion likes people who do hard work and God appreciates those kinds of people" (male, aged 65)

Islam promotes healthy eating and not to eat to excess, and to look after one's body by way of exercising. The following male respondent also echoes the same message, the importance of exercising and, in his opinion, the many opportunities that exist to encourage healthy behaviours and the importance of educating individuals of the benefits,

> "People should be encouraged to exercise where people should be educated about the importance of exercise so there is a need for awareness. There is no cultural barrier for doing any exercises, we have many opportunities for doing exercise if we have the will then we have no problem. There is no religious restrictions in exercising but our religion likes those people who are hardworking" (male, aged 65)

The next respondent talked about getting healthy messages across to individuals. One main stumbling block in Pakistan is the diversity in belief, from one spectrum of beliefs to another, from liberal families who actively encourage family members to get healthy to families that are ultra-conservative, who believe that going out in the community will only encourage mixing of the sexes. Islam is interpreted to the beliefs of elders and leaders, while individuals, particularly females, have little say,

> "We need to make aware and to tell them about the importance of exercise. There is no cultural barriers but you can say to some extent that people like my age do not like to go for exercise" (male, aged 63)

As highlighted through earlier comments, access to healthcare professionals is expensive, as the majority of doctors charge fees to see patients, usually 500 rupees. In addition to this, there are fees for tests and, if need be, for medications. A number of respondents believed that healthcare professionals should inform people about diseases. This is seen as essential in a developing country like Pakistan, especially advice on antenatal, postnatal and child well-being,

> "People can be encouraged through teaching them the importance of exercising and they should try and provide the facilities and the doctors should tell the people so to avoid diseases" (male, aged 60)

In contrast to the views of some male respondents cited above, the experiences of female respondents were wholly different. Cultural beliefs were dominant and the protection of females is seen as maintaining one's izzat (honour). The following female remarks on the barriers or restrictions placed on females that prevent them from going to a fitness centre, even though, like in her situation, she would benefit from attending. It is important to remember that restrictions are not only placed on young females, but older females also,

> "If someone goes outside of the home to a fitness centre than there are restrictions from our religion, but if we do exercises at home or walk outside then there are no restrictions" (female, aged 61)

When going to the gym was not an option for females, they were allowed to do what they could at home. This mainly took the form of daily household chores or doing the gardening. This respondent believed that there were no religious restrictions,

> "We have cultural barriers in our society but we can do it at home. In our religion it's not forbidden" (female, aged 60)

Again, reiterating the family and community life in parts of Pakistan,

> "I think someone my age if they do the housework it's easier for them I would encourage them to do. We have cultural barriers, to some extent I think in our religion there are cultural barriers for ladies, it's hard to go to any fitness centre" (female, aged 65)

Another female was more optimistic about change in long-held beliefs opening up to new possibilities,

> "There are religious restrictions about not being able to go to a fitness centre, but there's nothing about walking or doing exercises at home. To some extent there are cultural barriers but now this is going to change" (female, aged 62)

For the individual's well-being, it is paramount to have genuine choice and the ability to exercise it. In order to feel part of the biraderi and to subscribe to its ethos and values, one has to fully believe in its existence. For some females, they feel isolated from the outside world. Fitness centres not only provide health benefits to the dedicated attendee, but they also allow ladies to mix in a social context. Just being able to have a chit chat at the gym, to talk about family matters, worries, concerns and upbeat stories all clearly have a mental benefit on individuals. The point to remember is that females have few outlets to get away from the home unescorted, or indeed from the household chores of family life, to shop in the bazaar or to simply have tea in a cafe alone. In addition, and in the wider context, this is an illustration of generational tensions between the young and the old and between siblings and their parents. The willingness to change from perceived behaviours is enormously difficult for most families to comprehend and it needs a cultural shift.

Cultural barriers

Fitness centres and gyms were seen by many females as male-dominated spaces, thus inappropriate for females to attend unless there were separate provisions for male and females. The 'environment' of the gym was seen by some older females as not good. It was also about the fear of not knowing what happens behind the closed doors of the gym, but the main concern expressed was an inappropriate mixing of the sexes,

> "It is not a good environment for Asian women, there are men present in such places and women wear inappropriate clothes. I would let my daughters go to a women-only fitness centre where the staff are women and there are no men present then I do not mind. I am a modern woman I do not want to hold my daughters back from living a modern life, but they must know their limits" (female, aged 51)

The separate provision for males and females was seen as a solution to overcoming cultural barriers that could allow mothers and daughters to attend without the fear of repercussions from the biraderi,

> "There could be fitness centre just for women so they can wear whatever they want to and not feel awkward. Asian women especially might be reluctant to wear swimming costumes and leggings in front of men and there should be women-only swimming classes. There aren't any religious restrictions on exercise, everyone should exercise as long as women, especially Pakistani, are modestly dressed or in a women-only environment where they can wear exercise gear so they should exercise more" (female, aged 72)

Similar suggestions were raised by the following female respondent, who had the idea of 'family' type gyms, where mothers could take their younger children with them,

> "I and other Pakistani women would feel comfortable exercising and 'dancing' in a female Pakistani environment. People would exercise more if classes were local and free even if only once a week for an hour. Children should be allowed to attend as well so the women can come to the classes in the first place" (female, aged 55)

A typical day

To illustrate how cultural values and traditions play a dominant role in the lives of males and females, prompts were used to gain insights of individuals and their daily lives through exploring one's daily routine. For example, how they spent their day in general and any interests and hobbies pursued.

For retired male respondents, much of the time was spent either socialising or spending time at home. An early morning walk was the main activity preferred by male respondents, especially during the hot summer months,

> "I get up early in the morning and go out for a walk for about half an hour then I come back and do breakfast then I do the housework and I sometimes go out to meet someone in the evenings then I come back home" (male, aged 65)

Another reason to get up early in the morning was to read the Fajr Namaz (first prayer of the day) and this was followed by a stroll. The interesting habit was that male respondents went for a walk and then returned home to have breakfast. For most, this was a habit of lifetime, getting up early in the morning, usually 5am, reading the Namaz, followed by breakfast before setting off to work,

> "I get up early in the morning and after my prayers I go for some exercise, then I spend some time at home, after that I go outside to do some work, in the afternoon I meet my friends" (male, aged 65)

Others combined two things together, namely walking to the mosque to read the daily prayers. There are a large number of mosques in Mirpur and most attendees walk less than two hundred yards to pray. After prayers, male respondents returned home to have breakfast and those who could would read the daily newspaper, while those who could not read watched the daily news headlines on television,

> "I go to the mosque for prayers then walk around for about half an hour then I return home for my breakfast. After that I read the newspaper and

> spend time at home, then I go to my business office and sit over there or sometimes I go to meet my friends" (male, aged 60)

Socialising with friends and relatives was an important daily activity for male respondents. Much of the afternoon was set aside to meet up with friends, especially those who had come from afar and particularly those coming from the UK.

An important time for the household is when friends and family come to stay. Meeting and greeting is an important phase of creating and maintaining family bonds, thus considerable time and effort is put into making this as right as possible. This keeps older men busy and mobile, especially when organising sightseeing tours for visitors. There are a number of parks, forts and areas of natural beauty, most of which involve lengthy walks.

This was in contrast to the experience of many older females, where the division of labour was clearly evident. Most of the day was spent within the home and the main activity was cooking, preparing and serving food. Again, when friends and relatives came to stay, this only increased the amount of cooking and cleaning the woman had to do. If the family had a daughter-in-law(s), then they would do the bulk of the work under the supervision of the mother-in-law,

> "Most of the time I spend at home during the day time but sometimes I go outside. In the evening I do only the routine housework and spend time with my grandson and my daughter" (female, aged 61)

Similarly, another older female echoed,

> "Normally during the daytime I do the housework" (female, aged 65)

The experiences of most Pakistani women cut across sect and caste lines. A 'normal' day for older Pakistani women is cooking and doing the household chores. Friends and family who visited only led to more work, preparing, cooking and serving food followed by washing-up. Few households have a dishwasher, so it is a chore that is done by hand. Although an increasing number of households have access to tap water, there are still those who have to fetch water from a community well, often some distance away,

> "During the day I only do the routine work after that I do the housework" (female, aged 62)

A typical evening

For most respondents (both male and female) the evening was spent at home or, as discussed earlier, going for a stroll to the park or to the bazaar or greeting friends and family is a favourite pastime.

"In the evenings I sit with my old friends who live nearby" (male, aged 63).

If nothing special was planned, time was spent watching television, the favourite programmes being dramas. The content and the storylines nearly always evolved around community and family matters, especially finding a partner for the son or daughter; the search for love and upholding the family values were the usual topics of great interest. Watching dramas was also downtime after another busy day,

> "I watch TV regularly then I eat dinner and go to bed early" (male, aged 65)

Similarly,

> "In the evening I watch TV, I also do some studying" (male, aged 65)

Mode of travel

The most preferred method of getting from one place to another was 'walking', as some respondents would walk several miles to see friends and family.

> "When I go to town or go to visit my friends then I mostly go on foot when I have to go far away then I use the car. Mostly I walk because it is good for your health" (male, aged 65)

Walking was especially preferred during the cooler months of spring and autumn. The hot summers of Pakistan meant that few individuals went out in the basking sunshine, particularly during the midday sun. In fact, few individuals ventured out even in the car because of the heat and only made the essential journey. The following respondent was typical of many when he said,

> "When I go out to town mostly I walk and when I go far then I go by bus. Mostly I walk daily because I like to walk I do not use the car" (male, aged 65)

Again, distance walking was common for most and a good way of getting some exercise at the same time. However, walking had its perils, as the temptation to stop at the many street traders selling fast foods was a realistic outcome. For those relatives living further away, there was no option but to catch the bus,

> "I walk regularly about one to two miles. I never use the car for my travels when I go to town and when I go far I use the bus" (male, aged 63)

Using the car as a mode of travel was infrequent and, for some, 'rare',

> "I walk when I have to go to the town or when visiting friends. Very rarely I use the car or the taxi" (female, aged 62)

'Visiting' relatives is a favourite pastime for Pakistanis, as is attending festivals. Events like weddings, births and deaths are well-attended, often hundreds of people gathering for these events; they are communal events. It helps bind the community and also they are a good way of transferring values and traditions to younger people.

At the same time, they can be useful places for transferring information, particularly on health. For example, Pakistani men can often be heard talking about diabetes and heart disease and discussions often stem from an individual who has been diagnosed with the condition. It is a good place to share information and give advice to both sufferers and non-sufferers alike, for example the early symptoms, when to see the GP or, in more urgent cases, when to go to the hospital as an emergency case, especially those who have heart problems. Much of this is a public discussion and those with some health knowledge are encouraged to share their thoughts. It is a useful place for all to share their experiences, both good and bad.

Ways of encouraging communities to live healthily

One of the specific recommendations made by respondents was the lack of appropriate health information which could help individuals to learn about physical activity and its benefits,

> "We should make special times or we have to arrange special programmes to encourage people to walk or run" (male, aged 65)

Suggestions from participants appear to be attainable, for example health messages that encourage individuals to go for a walk, or to engage in other types of physical activity such as gardening,

> "If people think seriously about their health and if they get spare time. People should be encouraged to walk or if we make them aware about their health and the diseases that are caused this way" (male, aged 63)

Although going for a stroll is probably the main physical activity among older Pakistanis, some of the dangers are apparent, for example prolonged exposure to the sun. In the blistering hot summers of Pakistan, few journeys are made when the sun is at its highest point, and few are able to afford sun cream to protect oneself from skin cancer. While dehydration is a real problem for individuals, bottled water can be expensive (depending upon where you live) and few buy bottled water as they go out for a lengthy walk. The following respondent felt that he was in 'good health' and, when prompted about what he felt kept him in 'good health', he replied it was walking every day,

> "People are very lazy and they are not thinking about their health; if they did think and are aware of the importance of walking then this should encourage them to walk more" (male, aged 65)

Pakistan is a developing country and, although health facilities such as fitness centres are beginning to increase in numbers, they are still out of reach for many ordinary Pakistanis. Cost is an important consideration and instead every rupee is used to feed and clothe the family. A change of cultural attitudes and increase in health spending is the way forward,

> "If we are given more facilities…I would feel more comfortable or healthier about myself" (male, aged 65)

Similarly, another respondent echoed,

> "If people do exercise and there should be more health facilities like in the UK then I think it will be easier for us to live healthy. Or if my buying power increased because sometimes I am not able to eat what I like so that I can be healthier" (21: male, aged 63)

This respondent echoes a number of concerns, namely the need for more health facilities. As mentioned earlier, in Pakistan one must pay a fee to see a doctor (apart from Government-run health centres, which are free to the very poor). One must also be able to afford enough food to feed their families, and not overlooking the fact malnutrition is a major problem in parts of Pakistan.

CHAPTER EIGHT

ACCESS TO HEALTH INFORMATION AND KNOWLEDGE

The keys to promoting healthy behaviours are health messages that are understood by different groups in society. They have to be religiously and culturally sensitive; for example, attempting to increase physical activity among older Pakistani females, where the recommendation is to go jogging, are likely to fail because of cultural barriers within their own biraderi (kin) groups.

Tod et al. (2001) found that patient and community groups all had a lack of knowledge and awareness about the causes, treatments, and risks of heart disease. In reality, much of the health information, whether factually correct or not, is passed through extended kin network ties, especially among the older non-English speaking patients.

In a study by Ulvi et al. (2009) to determine baseline level awareness amongst a rural community, out of a sample of 300 only 129 (49%) of adults had any awareness of diabetes mellitus. They found that participants who had regular contact with health providers were more aware of diabetes and the associated risk factors than those who did not (71% v. 35%). They suggested raising public awareness of the disease through outreach programmes and mass media.

In developed countries, an increasing number of patients are accessing health-related information from the Internet; equally, health professionals are also using the Internet to seek information (Roscoe, 1998; Wilson, 1999). There are several reasons why patients are accessing the Internet; for example, to assume more responsibility for their health, but others could be forced to use the Internet because of lack of confidence in the healthcare system. Dolan (2003) found that the majority of patients (80%) preferred to access their GP as a source of obtaining health information, while accessing the Internet was the second most preferred method of accessing health information.

Health information was received from a variety of sources including health professionals, television, radio, newspapers, leaflets, friends and family and community networks. The preferred format of information received was dependent upon whether the individual could read. Illiteracy is the main barrier to accessing health information. Although respondents had a 'preferred' method of receiving health information, they were always open to new ways of understanding health messages,

> "The TV and magazines, my colleagues and wife" (male, aged 52)

Healthcare professionals

Health care professionals are the first point of reference for accurate and reliable health advice for respondents. Although there are many medical surgeries in Mirpur, most are privately owned and thus charge a 'fee' to see a doctor; as discussed earlier, this means most Pakistanis have no choice but to attend a government-run surgery. Private-run surgeries do provide free services to the most deprived of patients, for example the 'fee' is waived' and the patient buys the medications prescribed. Advice from healthcare professionals was, on many occasions, used with advice given by other professionals and lay people.

> "My GP gives me health advice as does the nurse. I watch --- --- (Asian channel) they have health programmes" (female, aged 56)

Health centres

Health centres are a lifeline to most families in Pakistan. Most are able to obtain free advice from professionals at health centres. Advice on contraception, child ailments and well-being are accessed by many Pakistanis. Although males attend health centres, they do so at different times.

Most attendees are women and health centres crucially provide protected space from the husband and other male relatives. It is a place where females can talk openly and freely with nurses on any issue or concern they may have. They provide a respite to females and may be only the few occasions when the female ventures out of the family household. The benefits of health centres are obvious to those who are literate and those with limited literacy skills,

> "I can learn of health issues through conferences or through listening on audio-taping or through nurses who come to us to inform us about health issues. We can learn through our doctors and nurses and through health

> centres as well, but doctors are too busy to help people and there needs to be more health centres to inform people" (male, aged 65)

Interestingly, health centres are also seen by individuals as a meeting place, to have a 'get together' and talk about concerns and worries, as well 'good feel' stories about successes in one's family. Generally, the 'ups and downs' of life,

> "I would like to receive information in the post. At the centres at the surgery. Seminars are good, you get to meet and see new and old friends" (male, aged 57)

The advice offered by health centres is crucial to improving the lives of ordinary Pakistanis. Health centres also provide community visits and these are particularly important to those living in remote villages in parts of Pakistan, where the nearest health centre may take two hours to reach. This can be practically impossible for the female, especially if she has young children to care for and travelling on the bus escorted by a male relative is unheard of even in present-day Pakistan. Cost of travelling to the health centre is another important factor; although travel may appear 'cheap' to affluent families, for those who are struggling on very limited incomes a 100-rupee bus ride can mean the difference between feeding a family of six and attending a health centre,

> "There are many ways to get to know about health issues like through the media or through your doctor or through your health centre. From our doctor and we have the lady health visitors in the villages and health centres we can go there for learning purposes" (female, aged 65)

Health centre teams are sensitive to the needs of local people and communities and they are 'trusted' by male relatives in that they provide a genuine service. Space is provided by the community leaders for healthcare teams to set up camp for the day and females are 'free' to attend; if resources allow, refreshments are provided especially during the hot summer months. One-to-one advice is followed up by lectures to the whole group of women, especially on contraception and how to look after oneself during pregnancy, childbirth as well as advice on symptoms on post-natal depression. Much of this community-led advice leads to females 'looking after one another', especially during pregnancy,

> "I learn about health issues through our doctors or through our health centres or if there are special health teams that can teach people about health issues then this will make it easy for me" (female, aged 63)

Similarly another said,

> "Through the media, but there should be special teams to make people aware or through our doctors or health centres if we keep in touch with them" (female, aged 62)

Television

Television and satellite channels are an excellent way of delivering health messages to large groups of people. For those who are literate, they would access both Asian and English channels to access health information. However, those who had issues around literacy, health channels provide an invaluable service where individuals can listen to the discussion instead. Information is provided in an easy to understand fashion and in layperson's terms; for example, symptoms of diabetes are a regular discussion on television,

> "There should be more television programmes about health in Urdu for people who cannot read especially in Asian channels like ---- and ---- TV" (female, aged 66)

To do this effectively, one needs to understand the needs of its viewers. Asian channels in particular do this adequately. They take into account the reviews provided by viewers and, if need be, change the format of the show,

> "I like listening to Asian radio stations and watching TV programmes as well. I watch '----- ----' on ---- ----- they have a regular slot for a doctor and he always talks about interesting health topics" (female, aged 51)

Similarly, another female respondent expressed her preference,

> "I like TV programmes and radio shows" (female, aged 61)

It was important to viewers that information was relevant and, at the same time, delivered in an interesting way, especially to viewers who have literacy issues,

> "I like to learn about health issues from TV programmes, it makes them more understandable and it is interesting to watch them. If I had a leaflet or a booklet I could read some of it but not all. I understand English very well, but it is not so easy reading it" (female, aged 57)

Again,

> "I like watching health programmes best so I like receiving health information via the TV" (female, aged 54)

It is interesting to note that the main language of communication on television is Urdu rather than a particular dialect. In Pakistan, there can be a hundred dialects spoken depending upon the particular geographical location or village in Pakistan.

Radio

There are many radio stations in Pakistan that cater for the needs of a very diverse population. Although the main medium of communication is Urdu, the official language of Pakistan, there are a large number of dialects that are spoken in Pakistan and radio stations cater for the needs of its listeners. It was interesting to note how respondents used the many different forms of media to learn about health issues,

> "I like booklets and TV programmes. I also sometimes listen to the radio especially ---- Radio" (female, aged 56)

The key message here is that culturally appropriate information is invaluable if delivered in a way that meets the needs of communities.

Newspapers

There were major differences between those respondents who could read and those who had to rely on family and friends for information. By far, it was preferable if the individual was in a position to read about health issues themselves. Published health stories in national newspapers were a common choice for such respondents,

> "I like to read the newspaper the most" (male, aged 56)

In Pakistan, there are a number of national newspapers but also a number of local and regional newspapers, again catering for a diverse population. Popular stories include health matters and local developments,

> "I like reading Urdu papers" (male, aged 54)

Similarly, again,

> "I like to read so a booklet or magazine is ideal" (female, aged 49)

Friends and family

For all respondents in this research, information received from educated or literate members of the family was invaluable. Siblings delivered health information in a way that was easy to understand.

However, one disadvantage to siblings translating health information is that there is the real possibility that it could be lost in translation. It is in effect a lay person's interpretation of health conditions and advice and there is no way of establishing whether this information is translated correctly or not. Siblings also ensured that only the relevant information was given to parents and grandparents who were not in a position to do so themselves,

> "My daughters tell me about health issues and so do my friends" (female, aged 62)

Again,

> "My daughter often tells me about health issues, my GP and health centre are very good as well. I can read English so I learn from leaflets and watch health programmes" (female, aged 54)

Again,

> "My GP sometimes gives me health advice but not very often. I usually talk to friends about health issues and if we have a health problem our daughters usually find out about it for us from books and leaflets" (female, aged 55)

In a developing country like Pakistan, information about health prevention is priceless. In a country where there is no welfare benefits or sickness benefits, looking after oneself especially if one is breadwinner becomes even more essential.

Community Networks

All information becomes available in the community domain, whether it is factual, incorrect or just gossip. Community networks are powerful networks which determine the lives of individuals and families alike. Any bit of information is shared within the community network and they are very useful in getting the message across. For example, in Pakistan vegetable ghee was the preferred choice among both the affluent and poorer families, and community networks ensured the negative impact of using vegetable ghee on one's health were explained to families. Similarly, community networks ensured the health messages regarding cutting down on salt were explained to individuals and families. In this sense, Pakistan has the advantage that healthcare professionals can use community networks to put their message across. There are direct beneficial outcomes for individuals,

> "I learn about health issues through our doctors or through the conferences (village gathering arranged by health professionals) but we go infrequently to see the doctor or the health centre" (female, aged 61)

Language barriers

A theme that runs throughout the book is literacy, where language acts as a barrier to accessing information. For example, in relation to health, the following respondent explains that there is little point in publishing health leaflets because there are people who are unable to read that information,

> "I would like there to be a health information shop with people who speak Punjabi who can give information about any health issues or problems I or my friends have. The health centres are usually full of leaflets but what use are they if you have trouble reading English and Urdu? It is better to talk to someone face-to-face" (female, aged 55)

Again,

> "I would like to get health information through representatives like yourself as you have come or there should be special programmes so we can receive information about health research" (male, aged 63)

Despite technological advances, for example easier access to the telephone, email and social media sites, older Pakistanis and those with limited language skills rely heavily on face to face contact. However, realising that, at times, this is not possible, respondents in this position rely heavily on siblings to translate information,

> "I prefer to listen to or watch health programmes, there is no point sending me leaflets or booklets I cannot read them and they end up in the bin!" (male, aged 72)

Again,

> "I like to learn about health information from people not from books as I cannot read. So my GP or friends are who I would go to for health information" (female, aged 62)

Receiving health information: Audio tape

Respondents made a number of recommendations for getting around language barriers, for example having information on audio tape/CD. Audio tape allows individuals to listen to information at a time that is most suitable to them. For example, during the evening when all the family has gathered together they can sit and listen to the commentary. Most families in Pakistan either own a tape recorder/CD player or have access to one and is a good way of getting health messages into homes,

> "I would like to receive health information through audio taping or there should be special teams like yourselves to inform people" (male, aged 65)

Another method suggested by some respondents was videotaping or on a CD in the form of a short film. This is particularly useful because individuals can see visually the information presented to them and, if this is backed up with support from health care professionals, then this could prove,

> "The best way for receiving health information for illiterate people is through videotaping and the second way is through doctors, nurses and through such interviews as well" (female, aged 60)

Issues affecting Mirpuris

We had a number discussions with participants about the state of their health and whether they thought they were healthy or otherwise. Interestingly, all respondents compared their health status to when they were younger. Conditions such as cancer, diabetes and high blood pressure have become prevalent in Mirpur, as have increasing cases of hepatitis B and C,

> "The health of the Pakistanis here in Mirpur is not good as compared to earlier, now people are suffering from many diseases like blood pressure and hepatitis B and C and also because of the water we are using and our food as well" (male, aged 65)

Respondents also compared the status of health to developed countries,

"The health of the Pakistanis overall is not to the satisfied level in this period of time people have many diseases and the health facilities have not improved like when compared to the advanced countries" (male, aged 65)

Environmental Factors

Pakistan is seriously confronted by many complex and difficult environmental challenges related to air, water, soil, forests and food issues, including climate change. The close link between environment and health is yet to be understood. The annual cost of environmental gradation in Pakistan has been estimated to be around US $4bn or at least 6% of the country's GDP. Up to 35% of the burden of disease is attributable to environmental hazards and risk factors and most of this burden is preventable (Khan et al., 2010).

This is similar to environmental issues and concerns were expressed by respondents who believed that they have a negative impact on people's lives. Issues such as heavy traffic in built-up areas like Mirpur were seen as negatives to health outcomes, particularly in the central areas of the district. Many of these issues are applicable to any industrialised city across the globe.

There is a growing concern that future development planning of the district needs to take into account issues such as heavy traffic that could be re-routed out away from the district. For many residents, the preference was always for greener spaces in the district such play areas and parks allowing residents to get away for the hustle and bustle of living in a major city,

"The important issues affecting health here (Mirpur) are polluted water, heavy traffic and lack of trees" (male, aged 62)

Similarly,

"We use impure water and we have pollution we have heavy traffic and very old transport so all of these issues affect our health" (male, aged 65)

Again,

"The important issues affecting us that we have dust here and we need to improve water and pollution as well these are the issues affecting our health" (male, aged 65)

Pollution appears to be a major concern for residents of the district and the push towards cleaner air and living is seen as a basis for healthy improvement,

> "We use impure water and we have pollution we have heavy traffic and very old transport so all of these issues affect our health" (male, aged 65)

All of the above environmental concerns were termed as 'difficult issues' by this respondent. However, there have been advances made in providing cleaner and sufficient water to residents of the district; many residents are able to afford to have a tanker deliver fresh, clean water to their home, often on a weekly basis. However, major problems in relation to the infrastructure remain,

> "Now people suffer from many types of diseases because of the difficult issues" (male, aged 63)

The overriding consensus among participants was one for continual improvement and exploring new ways of how best this could be achieved,

> "We should try to control all the things affecting our health and try to look at ways through which we can improve our health" (male, aged 65)

This covered a whole series of issues including environmental, changes in dietary habits and increasing physical activity among all groups in society,

> "Health can be improved by educating people about diseases caused by our lifestyle like our laziness, not working or exercising and not eating fresh foods and we should prevent ourselves from drinking fizzy drinks only then we can improve our health and we can live a better life" (female, aged 61)

There are other issues that have an important bearing on one's health status. For example, family and biraderi (kin) life plays an important role in the lives of individuals. For many, the biraderi can be a source of great emotional comfort and support, but for others it can be the basis of tension and difference. All individuals are governed by it and its rules and practices; adherence is seen as a prerequisite for being a valued member.

Preference for Pakistan or England in terms of lifestyle? (Din, 2008)

In my earlier book (Din, 2008), questions were centred around comparing the lifestyle of Pakistanis before migrating to the UK.

Dietary habits prior to migration

Migration had a major impact on the food consumption of Pakistanis through changes in dietary behaviour and availability and affordability of Western foods. Researchers have argued that food is most often the last item to be changed after migration (Mennell et al., 1992: Murcott, 1983).

Research has shown that Asian women had a variable dietary experience before their arrival in the UK (Eaton et al., 1984); but, as we will see, this also applied to the dietary habits of men. As you will note, the following elderly female enjoyed eating fatty foods such as paranthas, which have a high content of ghee. Foods that were high in fat content such as vegetable ghee, lassi and makka (corn roti) were seen as 'healthy foods'. They were foods that gave one strength, especially for day labourers (the majority of the respondents interviewed belonged to this group). Now these foods are seen to be unhealthy by health professionals. It is among this group that changing attitudes remains difficult. She also remarks that she 'never had fruit' before she came to the UK,

> "I ate paranthas with every meal. My husband may God bless him he was a man who enjoyed food we used to laugh and eat. I cooked with ghee, made eggs, had loads of pickles and never had fruit" (woman, aged 68)

Another female mentioned that during her teenage years she enjoyed eating batai (Asian sweets) and deep-fried savoury snacks,

> "I came to England when I was just out of my teenage years and have lived most of [my] adult life here. When I was in Pakistan I remember it as being very happy time in my life. I used to eat lots of sweets, batai (Asian sweets), honey bees (Asian boiled sweets) dried fruit and fruit juices and cake. I used to eat a lot of savoury snacks, samosas and deep-fried pasties every day. My parents really spoiled me and I was given any food I wanted" (woman, aged 49)

This equally applied to male respondents. Like most of the female respondents, their food also contained high levels of ghee, particularly in cooking, and sugary drinks,

> "I ate a lot of curries made out of ghee and I drank a lot of mango juice. I used to normally just eat and sleep it off due to the weather" (man, aged 57)

Most respondents had limited foods before their migration to the UK; this was soon to change, as the following respondent explained,

> "Meat, vegetables and fruit, lentils and vegetables are the staple diet in Pakistan and chicken and lamb are served twice a week if you have the money. In the mornings I used to eat pakoras with milk lassi. I would eat a vegetable curry at lunchtime and have curried eggs or chicken in the evenings. I used to eat a lot of apples, oranges and mangoes in Pakistan. I would eat pakoras every day I would buy them from stalls in the bazaar (market)" (man, aged 54)

Similarly another female said,

> "In Pakistan I ate only fresh food, freshly slaughtered chicken and lamb and fresh vegetables and fruit. All the food in Pakistan is local and there are no imports especially the village that I am from they probably have not seen strawberries or avocados either. I used to eat chapattis and curry three times a day sometimes chicken and dal or cauliflower or some other vegetable. I would eat mangoes a lot and have batai (Asian sweets) a lot, batai is regularly served with tea and is not a luxury as it is in England" (woman, aged 51)

The following respondent's dietary intake was typical of most respondents before their migration,

> "I remember eating dal (lentils) a lot of the time. We used to eat chillies crushed with coriander and onion curry with chapatti a lot. Butter and ghee was used on chapattis a lot and spinach is eaten widely. I used to drink a lot of lassi (milky Asian drink); young men are given it often to make them strong. On some days I would just eat a watery curry with ginger, garlic and aniseed, almonds grounded were added if you were lucky. The food I ate in Pakistan was simple, plain and functional" (man, aged 72)

Similarly, the following respondent revealed her food consumption prior to migration and how vividly she remembers this, in particular recalling that she ate fresh vegetables, milk and chicken,

> "In Pakistan I ate a lot of fruit and vegetable curries. I used to eat mangoes every day, two or three at a time. We would have a lot of cauliflower, kerala (bitter grout) and okra curries. I used to eat meat twice a week. Everything is fresh in Pakistan, the chickens used to live in a small hut outside the house. The milk was fresh everything was pure and healthy. I used to especially like drinking lassi (Pakistani milk drink)" (woman, aged 53)

Equally, respondents ate much more fruit and vegetables before their migration and consumed less meat; this was not out of choice, but often the result of limited income where meat was expensive to purchase. This suggests that migration plays an important role in the dietary behaviours of British Pakistanis,

> "I ate a lot of fruit and vegetables. Lentils were eaten a lot and dried chickpeas and red kidney bean curry. I would eat a lot of spinach, cauliflower, tomatoes and moolie dishes. I ate chapatti three times a day in Pakistan we did not have bread. Rice was served once a week and it usually had moonga dal (lentils) inside it. Chicken was cooked once a week and considered a treat. I would eat boiled eggs with my evening meal the food was basic but healthy" (man, aged 56)

Interestingly, all the respondents thought they were healthier when they lived in Pakistan (prior to migration) than in the UK. What comes out consistently is that, in Pakistan (although most were in their youth years), they had plenty of fresh air, exercise (often through working in manual labour) and fresh food and ingredients compared to consuming much more salt and fat in their diet in the UK. Although the following respondent would like to move back to Pakistan, his son's work keeps him in England,

> "I was healthier in Pakistan because I walked more and ate less fattening [food]. I think that the angina has been caused by too much fat and salt in my diet. I would not move back to Pakistan. I get a pension here, my son makes a good living. I would not move back home just to eat more healthy" (man, aged 72)

Moving to a cleaner, social environment was a positive incentive for one lady who wished to move back to Pakistan. At the same time, she realised her diet would only be better. A number of respondents were reminiscing about the 'good old days' of a healthy diet in Pakistan. Although this was the case for some (among the more affluent), for most who belonged to the lower caste their diet was very limited. The staple everyday foods were flour (consumed through chapattis or roti), salam (curry); they nearly always had lentils, pulses and vegetables (such as spinach and cauliflower), which were much cheaper than meat and chicken. Fruit was also consumed, especially mangoes, melon and watermelon, as these were plentiful. A clean social environment was important,

> "I lived a more healthy life in Pakistan and the food I ate was fresh and healthy. I would not mind moving back to Pakistan, I would be away from all the rotten meat smells from the incinerator and my diet would be better" (woman, aged 53)

However, things have gradually changed in Mirpur,

> "I lived more healthily in Pakistan even with the changes in Pakistan and the imported Western foods. It is still healthier especially in the villages like Mirpur which are virtually untouched by the Western lifestyle and food choices. I would move back to Pakistan as my friends and relatives are there. I would move back to be healthy as in ten years ago. I think Pakistani food will be overtaken by all the imported Western food so there is no escape wherever I go" (man, aged 56)

A better or much easier lifestyle was another factor that would influence people as to whether they thought living in the UK was better than Pakistan in terms of better diet and lifestyle. This woman felt more 'relaxed' in Pakistan, with a better, warmer climate all year round and where all the food was cooked at home,

> "I was healthier in Pakistan, the lifestyle there is more relaxed. There is fresh air and healthy food all of which is home cooked and good for you" (woman, aged 55)

The majority of respondents said they 'overate' once they arrived in the UK. They had all the foods they had in Pakistan (including meat, chicken, fruit and vegetables), but also Western foods, for example cakes, biscuits, chocolates, fish and chips – foods that were considered as 'luxury' foods by the early settlers. All of these were readily available to them upon their migration in the late 1950s and early 1960s,

> "I ate more healthily in Pakistan because the food was fresher. I also had no biscuits or fizzy drinks there as they are considered luxuries and only given on special occasions to guests or at weddings. In England I eat biscuits every day, they are not healthy but I am thankful I can afford them and I make a good living in England. I would not move back to Pakistan, the food is healthy but I would miss my 'luxury' food like fizzy pop and the food in England is quick to prepare; it might be unhealthy and less fresh, but quick to prepare" (woman, aged 51)

This was an important period because, particularly for men, it changed their attitudes towards diet and what they would consume later (and the period before their wives arrived in the UK).

> "I was healthy in Pakistan when I came to England I became unhealthy because I overate. I was overwhelmed by all the food I was able to afford. My overeating caused me health problems with my heart, it was a wake-up call for me and now I am healthier again. The diet in Pakistan is naturally healthy, people eat healthy food sometimes out of necessity because they cannot afford meat every night and have vegetables instead. Without

realising it, the people in Pakistan have a good healthy diet" (man, aged 54)

Healthy eating: Comparing Pakistan and UK present opinion

This research prompted respondents to compare life in Pakistan to the UK. Many respondents in this study had relatives living in the UK who frequently went back to Pakistan for holidays and family functions such as births, marriages and funeral. Stories about life in the UK are exchanged with relatives in Pakistan. Storytelling is an integral part of Pakistani life, and stories about changes in dietary habits is topical especially during mealtimes. Concerns around the frequency of consuming fast foods and takeaways has become the main focus of discussions, as are the negatives of leading a sedentary lifestyle.

Being healthy was the desired goal for many, and to stay fit and healthy for as long as possible in order to contribute services to everyday family and biraderi life. Being healthy also allowed one to be independent and mobile and, hopefully, free from debilitating conditions such as diabetes, which is rife among the Pakistani population. Those visiting Pakistan from the UK invariably compared their lifestyle to those in Pakistan, for example the frequency of consuming frozen foods in the UK compared to eating fresh, locally produced foods in Pakistan,

> "I eat healthily here (Pakistan) better than in the UK; it's because we eat fresh fruits and vegetables, and the taste of foods is different and people mostly in the UK eat frozen foods. So I think it's better to live here than over there, but there are more facilities there in the UK and so people like to live in the UK. The health facilities are very good compared to Pakistan" (male, aged 60)

The above respondent remarks on the importance of 'very good' health facilities available in the UK. The NHS is a tower of strength to the nation providing free care at the point of delivery to all its citizens, irrespective of need. It provides essential care to individuals when they fall ill. Long-term conditions such as diabetes are managed through services provided by primary and secondary care, something which is unavailable in Pakistan except to the very few.

For others, they noticed that those arriving from the UK did less strenuous work than those living in Pakistan and that they appeared to be fitter and healthier. This was a personal judgement based on an individual's ailments,

> "I look at people coming from the UK then I think we are healthy because we do more hard work and environmentally this country is good" (male, aged 63)

Similarly, another male respondent said,

> "I think we are healthy here because it is naturally and environmentally good to live here, otherwise in England there are more facilities and more cleanliness as compared to Pakistan" (male, aged 65)

As discussed earlier, one of the ways of living healthier was walking rather than using the car or catching the bus, especially for shorter journeys,

> "They do not go for a walk and they mostly use the car or the bus, for these reasons I think people are healthier in Pakistan than England" (female, aged 65)

The following respondent listed a number of differences between Pakistan and the UK, the main being the hot weather in Pakistan and the availability of fresh produce,

> "We eat fresh food and we do hard work and we have the advantage of the weather as well so I can say we are more healthier as compared to the UK. They have better health facilities than in Pakistan, but we have the advantage of higher temperatures in the UK, the temperatures are low and in this way I feel more healthier" (male, aged 65)

Again,

> "To some extent I can say that the people are healthier here (Pakistan) than in the UK, it's because of the weather change here you have higher temperature than in the UK" (24: Female, Aged 61)

Although warmer temperatures (during the cooler months of spring) were generally seen as having a positive impact on the body, by contrast excessively hot weather during the summer was seen by some as being negative. For example, these negatives included an increase in ailments, having to pay extra for water and ice and higher electricity bills due to running extra fans and generators (those who could afford to install them in their house).

CHAPTER NINE

CONCLUSION: THE IMPORTANCE OF UNDERSTANDING INDIVIDUALS AND COMMUNITIES

A theme that reverberates throughout the book is the need to understand individuals and communities. In order to do this effectively, researchers need to be proactive and engage with communities in a meaningful way. Research that uses inductive research methods should be in a position to understand the needs of individuals. The skill and the ability to listen to the messages coming from communities is an essential prerequisite to achieving the above. Ethnic minority communities are not homogenous. There are major differences between the Indian, Pakistani and the Bangladeshis, but there are also differences within communities; for example, within the Pakistani communities, differences exist along the lines of sect, caste, and cultural, as well as normative differences. Health professionals who wish to target communities need to understand these differences in order to develop interventions that would be beneficial to individuals and communities.

Proficiency in language, whether this is in English or Urdu, has a negative impact on individuals' lives. In Pakistan, health information is written in Urdu; however, a sizeable minority of older Pakistanis are unable to read, thus they are unable to access the information. Instead, respondents preferred to receive information in alternative formats such as health programmes on the radio and television. What this shows is that a generic approach to putting health messages across as a whole may not be getting across to the very people that need it the most.

The lack of English language skills or not being able to read in their native language is equally a problem in the UK. For example, there are several hundred languages and dialects spoken in the UK. Providing translated information in all the different languages and costs involved can be substantial, as are providing interpreting services to institutions and, at the same time, having to provide culturally competent services and care.

A number of chapters in this book are devoted to helping researchers understand communities, particularly minority ethnic communities. Advice and practical tips discussed should help researchers go out into the community with some confidence. Researchers are constantly struggling to meet data collection goals. Recruiting for all intents and purposes is 'tough', even for the most dedicated and experienced of researchers. Being sent out into the community can prove to be a daunting task. Much of what happens 'out there' depends upon the knowledge and background of the researcher. If he/she approaches the task with an open approach, and one that involves meeting the community on 'its own turf', it will lead to constructive engagement and make recruitment much less daunting. There are many opportunities to 'meet the community', for example through festivals and melas, at community centres, places of worship and Sunday markets. One can do as much or as little as they want, but this activity involves a considerable amount of time to develop and act.

Community contacts can prove useful in this task, and elders and gatekeepers can act as an access point to a large number of participants. One must bear in mind that gatekeepers are regularly contacted by researchers to help them with recruiting 'hard to reach' individuals. Gatekeepers will help if they are in a position to and should not be expected to proactively recruit for researchers, but only give helpful pointers to aid recruitment.

It is stating the obvious, but if the researcher has recruited from a community setting, for example from a community centre, or needed the help of a gatekeeper, then they should be acknowledged. Further, once the data collection has finished, it is necessary to re-visit and provide an update and, of course, to deliver the final report once it is completed.

So what does the data reveal in this book? Namely, that getting the health message across to individuals and communities can be an uphill struggle for health professionals in terms of limiting dietary intake and increasing physical activity amongst all groups of society.

In this sample in Mirpur, Pakistan, the increased availability in fast foods and their relative cheapness has meant that many more individuals are having such foods on a regular basis rather than infrequently. The dietary habits of older Pakistanis have changed considerably since when they were younger, with a limited but healthy diet relying on fresh locally produced crops, fruit and vegetables coupled with plenty of hard work. A diet of high carb and high fat, takeaway foods such fried food, pizzas, fizzy drinks and sweet deserts have all but replaced their earlier healthier diet. This, for some Pakistanis, has had a major impact on their health status, for example the high incidences of diabetes and high blood pressure have affected most families in Pakistan. A message that is echoed by many Pakistanis is that "people should try to eat fresh food and try to avoid eating takeaways" (male, aged 63).

Those who had limited incomes in Pakistan consumed foods that were within their monthly budgets, mainly relying on vegetables and pulses to feed the family. Fast foods and fizzy drinks were consumed infrequently, normally on special occasions such as to celebrate a birth or marriage. If they had a sizeable plot of land, then they grew their own fruit and vegetables at home to feed the family; these were usually chillies, onions, potatoes, okra and cauliflower. This meant that, especially during the summer months, the family would have something to eat. The price of sugar, tea and milk has increased considerably in recent years, thus some went without such foods. Healthy eating was considered by most as a luxury and only within the budgets of more affluent families who could afford to have a varied and healthy diet.

Like changes in dietary habits, there have also been changes in the levels of physical activity. Many respondents reported that they engaged in some form of physical activity when they were younger, whether this was through work or their favourite pastimes such as attending to their large gardens. Walking everywhere was the norm, partly because of the unaffordability and costs of transport, and partly because of the good weather in Pakistan; walking to the bazaar or a relative's home was what everybody did. This continues on the whole today but the usage of buses and cars is increasing, particularly as one's health deteriorates. For most Pakistanis, the aim was "I like to walk and this encourages me and it is exercise as well. This is the easiest way for me to exercise" (male, aged 65).

BIBLIOGRAPHY

Afzal, M.N. and Naveed, M. (2004) Childhood obesity and Pakistan. Journal of the College of Physicians and Surgeons Pakistan, March 2004, vol./is. 14/3(189-192).

Akatsu, H. and Aslam, A. (1996) Prevalence of hypertension and obesity among women over age 25 in a low income area in Karachi, Pakistan. The Journal of the Pakistan Medical Association, September 1996, vol./is. 46/9(191-3).

Alam, S.E. (1998) Prevalence and pattern of smoking in Pakistan. J Pak Med Assoc. 1998 Mar;48(3):64-6.

Ali, S., Ara, N., Ali, A., Ali, B. and Kadir, M.M. (2008) Knowledge and practices regarding cigarette smoking among adult women in a rural district of Sindh, Pakistan. J Pak Med Assoc. 2008 Dec;58(12):664-7.

Ali, S., Khuwaja, A.K., Ali, T. and Hameed, R. (2009) Smokeless tobacco use among adult patients who visited family practice clinics in Karachi, Pakistan. J Oral Pathol Med. 2009 May;38(5):416-21.

Ali, S., Sathiakumar, N. and Delzell, E. (2006) Prevalence and socio-demographic factors associated with tobacco smoking among adult males in rural Sindh,Pakistan. Southeast Asian J Trop Med Public Health. 2006 Sep;37(5):1054-60.

Ali, Z., Ahmed, S.M., Nageen, A., Tanveer, M., and Sohrab, S. (2014) Obesity & Diabetes: An experience at a public sector tertiary care hospital. Pak J Med Sci. 2014 Jan;30(1).

Allen, S. (1971), New Minorities Old Conflicts: Asian and West Indian migrants in Britain, Random House, New York,

Anwar, M. (1995) 'New Commonwealth Migration to the UK', in Cohen, R. (ed.), Cambridge Survey of World Migration, Cambridge University Press, Cambridge.

—. (1998) Between Cultures, Continuity and Change in the lives of Young Asians, Routledge, London.

Arjunan, S.P., Bishop, N.C., Reischak-Oliveira, A. and Stensel, D.J. (2013) Exercise and coronary heart disease risk markers in South Asian and European men. Med Sci Sports Exerc. Jul;45(7):1261-8.

Aslam, F., Mahmud, H. and Waheed, A. (2004) Cardiovascular health behaviour of medical students in Karachi. J Pak Med Assoc. 2004 Sep;54(9):492-5.

Aurora, G. S. (1967) The New Frontiersmen: A Sociological Study of Indian Immigrants in the United Kingdom, Popular Parakashan, Bombay.

Bainey, K.R. and Jugdutt, B. (2009) Increased burden of coronary artery disease in South-Asians living in North America. Need for an aggressive management algorithm. Atherosclerosis. May;204(1):1-10.

Ballard, R. (ed.) (1994) Desh Pardesh: The South Asian Presence in Britain, Hurst, London.

Basit, T. (1997) Eastern Values; Western Milieu Identities and Aspirations of Adolescent British Muslim Girls, Ashgate Publishing, Aldershot.

Bile, K.M., Shaikh, J.A., Afridi, H.U. and Khan, Y. (2010) Smokeless tobacco use in Pakistan and its association with oropharyngeal cancer. East Mediterr Health J. 2010;16 Suppl:S24-30.

Blackford, J. and Street, A. (2002) Cultural conflict: the impact of western feminism(s) on nurses caring for women of non-English speaking background. Journal of Clinical Nursing, 09 2002, vol./is. 11/5(664-71).

Blignault, I., Ponzio, V., Rong, Y., and Eisenbruch, M. (2008) A qualitative study of barriers to mental health services utilisation among migrants from mainland China in south-east Sydney. International Journal of Social Psychiatry, 03 2008, vol./is. 54/2(180-90).

Bowler, I.M. (1993) Stereotypes of women of Asian descent in midwifery: some evidence. Midwifery, 03 1993, vol./is. 9/1(7-16).

Braham, P. et al. (ed.) (1992) Racism, Anti-racism- Inequalities, opportunities and Policies, Newbury Park California, Sage in association with the Open University, London.

Brooks, N., Magee, P., Bhatti, G., Briggs, C., Buckley, S., Guthrie, S., Moltesen, H., Moore, C. and Murray, S. (2000) Asian patients' perspective on the communication facilities provided in a large inner city hospital. Journal of Clinical Nursing, 01 September 2000, vol./is. 9/5(706-712).

Brown, C. (1984) Black and White in Britain The Third PSI Survey, Policy Studies Institute, London.

Chan, Y.F. and Quine, S. (1997) Utilisation of Australian health care services by ethnic Chinese. Australian Health Review, vol./is. 20/1(64-77), 0156-5788.

Cortes, D.E., Drainoni, M.L., Henault, L.E. and Paasche-Orlow, M.K. (2010) How to achieve informed consent for research from Spanish-speaking individuals with low literacy: a qualitative report. Journal of Health Communication, 2010, vol./is. 15 Suppl 2 (172-82).

Costello, E., Kafchinski, M., Vrazel, J. and Sullivan, P. (2011) Motivators, barriers, and beliefs regarding physical activity in an older adult population. J Geriatr Phys Ther. 2011 Jul-Sep;34(3):138-47.

Cullingford, C. and Din, I. (2006) Ethnicity and Englishness: Personal Identities in a Minority Community. Cambridge Scholars Press, Newcastle.

Dahya, B. (1972-3) 'Pakistanis in England', New Community, No.2, pp. 25-33.

Davies, M.M. and Bath, P.A. (2001) The maternity information concerns of Somali women in the United Kingdom. Journal of Advanced Nursing, 10 2001, vol./is. 36/2(237-45), (2001 Oct).

Desai, R. (1963) Indian Immigrants in Britain, Oxford University Press, London.

Dodani, S., Mistry, R., Khwaja, A., Farooqi, M., Qureshi, R. and Kazmi K. (2004) Prevalence and awareness of risk factors and behaviours of coronary heart disease in an urban population of Karachi, the largest city of Pakistan: a community survey. J Public Health (Oxf). 2004 Sep;26(3):245-9.

Dunckley, M., Hughes, R., Addington-Hall, J. and Higginson, I.J. (2003) Language translation of outcome measurement tools: views of health professionals. International Journal of Palliative Nursing, 02 2003, vol./is. 9/2(49-55).

Easton, P., Entwistle, V.A. and Williams, B. (2013) How the stigma of low literacy can impair patient-professional spoken interactions and affect health: insights from a qualitative investigation. BMC Health Services Research, 2013, vol./is. 13/(319)

Farooq, M.U., Majid, A., Reeves, M.J. and Birbeck, G.L. (2009) The epidemiology of stroke in Pakistan: past, present, and future. Int J Stroke. 2009 Oct;4(5):381-9.

Fawwad, A., Alvi, S.F., Basit, A., Ahmed, K., Ahmedani, M.Y., Hakeem, R. (2013) Changing pattern in the risk factors for diabetes in young adults from the rural area of Baluchistan. J Pak Med Assoc. 2013 Sep;63(9):1089-93.

Fryer, P. (1984) Staying Power: The History of Black people in Britain, Pluto Press, London.

Fudge, N.W. and McKevitt, C. D. (2007) Involving older people in health research. Age & Ageing, 09 2007, vol./is. 36/5(492-500).

Galdas, P., Ratner, M., Pamela, Oliffe, A., and John, L. (2012) A narrative review of South Asian patients' experiences of cardiac rehabilitation. Journal of Clinical Nursing, 01 January 2012, vol./is. 21/1/2(149-159).

Gerrish, K. (2001) The nature and effect of communication difficulties arising from interactions between district nurses and South Asian patients and their carers. Journal of Advanced Nursing, 01 March 2001, vol./is. 33/5(566-574).

Gilani, S.I. and Leon, D.A. (2013) Prevalence and sociodemographic determinants of tobacco use among adults in Pakistan: findings of a nationwide survey conducted in 2012. Popul Health Metr. 2013 Sep 3;11(1):16.

Gill, P.S., Plumridge, G., Khunti, K. and Greenfield, K. (2013) Under-representation of minority ethnic groups in cardiovascular research: a semi-structured interview study. Family Practice, 04 2013, vol./is. 30/2(233-41).

Hanna, L., Hunt, C, Sonja, I., Bhopal, M. and Raj, S. (2012) Using the Rose Angina Questionnaire cross-culturally: the importance of consulting lay people when translating epidemiological questionnaires. Ethnicity & Health, 01 June 2012, vol./is. 17/3(241-251).

Hashmi, M., Khan, M. and Wasay, M. (2013) Growing burden of stroke in Pakistan: a review of progress and limitations. Int J Stroke. 2013 Oct;8(7):575-81.

Hayes, L., White, M., Unwin, N., Bhopal, R., Fischbacher, C., Harland, J. and Alberti, K.G. (2002) Patterns of physical activity and relationship with risk markers for cardiovascular disease and diabetes in Indian, Pakistani, Bangladeshi and European adults in a UK population. J Public Health Med. Sep;24(3):170-8.

Hipwell, A., Turner, A. and Barlow, J. (2008) 'We're not fully aware of their cultural needs': tutors' experiences of delivering the Expert Patients Programme to South Asian attendees. Diversity in Health & Social Care, 01 December 2008, vol./is. 5/4(281-290).

Holmes, C. (1991) A Tolerant Country? Immigrants, Refugees and Minorities in Britain, Faber, London.

Homer, C. (2000) Incorporating cultural diversity in randomised controlled trials in midwifery. Midwifery, 12 2000, vol./is. 16/4 (252-9).

Horne, M., Skelton, D.A., Speed, S. and Todd, C. (2013) Perceived barriers to initiating and maintaining physical activity among South Asian and White British adults in their 60s living in the United Kingdom: a qualitative study. Ethn Health. 2013;18(6):626-45.

Houston, A. M, and Cowley, S. (2003) Health needs assessment in the health visiting service and the impact on the ethnic community. International Journal of Nursing Studies, 01 2003, vol./is. 40/1(85-94).

Hui, E. and Devendra, D. (2010) Diabetes and fasting during Ramadan. Diabetes Metab Res Rev. 2010 Nov;26(8):606-10.

Hunt, S.M., and Bhopal, R. (2004) Self report in clinical and epidemiological studies with non-English speakers: the challenge of language and culture. Journal of Epidemiology & Community Health, 07 2004, vol./is. 58/7(618-22).

Hussain-Gambles, M., Atkin, K. and Leese, B. (2006) South Asian participation in clinical trials: the views of lay people and health professionals. Health Policy, 07 vol./is. 77/2(149-65).

Hussain-Gambles, M., Leese, B., Atkin, K., Brown, J., Mason, S. and Tovey, P. (2004) Involving South Asian patients in clinical trials. Health Technology Assessment (Winchester, England), 10, vol./is. 8/42(iii, 1-109).

Imam, S.F., Bhatti, A.M. and Lutufullah, N. (2000) Prevalence of obesity in south-east suburb of Lahore, Pakistan. Medical Forum Monthly, 2000, vol./is. 11/2(13-15).

Ishaque, A., Ahmad, F., Zehra, N. and Amin, H. (2012) Frequency of and factors leading to obesity and overweight in school children. J Ayub Med Coll Abbottabad. 2012 Apr-Jun;24(2):34-8.

Jafar, T.H. (2006) Women in Pakistan have a greater burden of clinical cardiovascular risk factors than men. Int J Cardiol. 2006 Jan 26;106(3):348-54.

Jafar, T.H., Islam, M., Poulter, N., Hatcher, J., Schmid, C.H., Levey, A.S. and Chaturvedi, N. (2005) Children in South Asia have higher body mass-adjusted blood pressure levels than white children in the United States: a comparative study. Circulation. 2005 Mar 15;111(10):1291-7.

Jafar, T.H., Jafary, F.H., Jessani, S. and Chaturvedi, N. (2005) Heart disease epidemic in Pakistan: women and men at equal risk. Am Heart J. 2005 Aug;150(2):221-6.

Jafar, T.H., Levey, A.S., Jafary, F.H., White, F., Gul, A., Rahbar, M.H., Khan, A.Q., Hattersley, A., Schmid, C.H. and Chaturvedi N. (2003) Ethnic subgroup differences in hypertension in Pakistan. J Hypertens. May; 21(5):905-12.

Jafar, T.H., Qadri, Z. and Chaturvedi, N. (2008) Coronary artery disease epidemic in Pakistan: more electrocardiographic evidence of ischaemia in women than in men. Heart. 2008 Apr;94(4):408-13. Epub 2007 Jul 23.

Kannon, C. T. (1978) Cultural adaptation of Asian immigrants-First and Second Generation, Greenford, The Author, 107 Hill Rise, Middlesex.

Khan, A., Huque, R., Shah, S.K., Kaur, J., Baral, S., Gupta, P.C., Cherukupalli, R., Sheikh, A., Selvaraj, S., Nargis, N., Cameron, I. and

Siddiqi, K. (2014) Smokeless Tobacco Control Policies in South Asia: A Gap Analysis and Recommendations. Nicotine Tob Res. 2014 Mar 10.

Khan, M.Z., Kazi, B.M., Bile, K.M., Magan, M. and Nasir, J.A. (2010) Environmental health needs and launching of an environmental health protection unit in Pakistan.East Mediterr Health J. 2010;16 Suppl:S69-75.

Khan, N.I., Naz, L., Mushtaq, S., Rukh, L., Ali, S. and Hussain, Z. (2009) Ischemic stroke: prevalence of modifiable risk factors in male and female patients in Pakistan. Pak J Pharm Sci. 2009 Jan;22(1):62-7.

Khan, V. S. (1979) (ed.) Migration and Social Stress: Mirpuris in Bradford, in Minority Families in Britain, Support and Stress, MacMillan, London.

Khuwaja, A.K. and Kadir, M.M. (2004) Smoking among adult males in an urban community of Karachi, Pakistan. Southeast Asian J Trop Med Public Health. 2004 Dec;35(4):999-1004.

Laws, M.B., Heckscher, R., Mayo, S.J., Li, W. and Wilson, I.B. (2004) A new method for evaluating the quality of medical interpretation. Medical Care, 01 2004, vol./is. 42/1(71-80).

Lee, T.S., Lansbury, G. and Sullivan, G. (2005) Health care interpreters: A physiotherapy perspective. Australian Journal of Physiotherapy, 2005, vol./is. 51/3(161-5).

Lewis, P. (1994) Islamic Britain, London, I.B Tavris and Co.

Lindesay, J., Jagger, C., Hibbett, M.J., Peet, S.M. and Moledina, F. (1997) Knowledge, uptake and availability of health and social services among Asian Gujarati and white elderly persons. Ethnicity & Health, 01 March 1997, vol./is. 2/1/2(59-69).

Lloyd C.E., Mughal, S., Stuart, J., O'Hare P. and Barnett A.H. (2006) Using self-complete questionnaires in a South Asian population with diabetes: problems and solutions. Diversity in Health & Social Care, December 2006, vol./is. 3/4(245-251).

Lowe, P., Griffiths, F. and Sidhu, R. (2007) 'I got pregnant, I was so like ... crying inside ...': experiences of women of Pakistani ancestry seeking contraception in the UK. Diversity in Health & Social Care, 01 March 2007, vol./is. 4/1(69-76).

Ludwig, A.F., Cox, P. and Ellahi, B. (2011) Social and cultural construction of obesity among Pakistani Muslim women in North West England. Public Health Nutr. 2011 Oct;14(10):1842-50.

Marlow, L.A., Robb, K.A., Simon, A.E., Waller, J. and Wardle, J. (2012) Awareness of cancer risk factors among ethnic minority groups in England. Public Health. 2012 Aug;126(8):702-9.

Marshall, S.L. and While, A. E. (1994) Interviewing respondents who have English as a second language: challenges encountered and suggestions for other researchers. Journal of Advanced Nursing, 03 1994, vol./is. 19/3(566-71).

Masood, C.T. and Afzal, W. (2013) Long-term complications of diabetes and co-morbidities contributing to atherosclerosis in diabetic population of Mirpur, Azad Kashmir. J Pak Med Assoc. 2013 Nov;63(11):1383-6.

Merchant, A., Husain, S.S., Hosain, M., Fikree, F.F., Pitiphat, W., Siddiqui, A.R., Hayder, S.J., Haider, S.M., Ikram, M., Chuang, S.K. and Saeed, S.A. (2000) Paan without tobacco: an independent risk factor for oral cancer. Int J Cancer. 2000 Apr 1;86(1):128-31.

Mygind, A., Kristiansen, M., Wittrup, I. and Nørgaard, L.S. (2013) Patient perspectives on type 2 diabetes and medicine use during Ramadan among Pakistanis in Denmark. Int J Clin Pharm. 2013 Apr;35(2):281-8.

Nadeem, M., Ahmed, S.S., Mansoor, S. and Farooq, S. (2013) Risk factors for coronary heart disease in patients below 45 years of age. Pak J Med Sci. 2013 Jan;29(1):91-6.

Nanan. D.J. (2002) The obesity pandemic-implications for Pakistan. The Journal of the Pakistan Medical Association, Aug 2002, vol./is. 52/8(342-346).

Nisar, N., Qadri, M.H., Fatima, K. and Perveen, S. (2008) Dietary habits and life style among the students of a private medical university Karachi. J Pak Med Assoc. 2008 Dec;58(12):687-90.

Phul, A., Bath, P.A. and Jackson, M.G. (2003) The provision of information by health promotion units to people of Asian origin living in the UK. Health Informatics Journal, 01 March 2003, vol./is. 9/1(39-56).

Qidwai, W., Saleheen, D., Saleem, S., Andrades, M. and Azam, S.I. (2003) Are our people health conscious? Results of a patients survey in Karachi, Pakistan. J Ayub Med Coll Abbottabad. 2003 Jan-Mar;15(1):10-3.

Råberg Kjøllesdal, M.K., Telle Hjellset, V., Bjørge, B., Holmboe-Ottesen, G. and Wandel, M. (2010) Barriers to healthy eating among Norwegian-Pakistani women participating in a culturally adapted intervention. Scand J Public Health. 2010 Nov;38(5 Suppl):52-9.

Rafique, G. and Khuwaja, A.K. (2003) Diabetes and hypertension: public awareness and lifestyle - findings of a health mela. J Coll Physicians Surg Pak. 2003 Dec;13(12):679-83.

Rahi, J.S., Manaras, I., Tuomainen, H., Lewando, S. and Hundt, G. (2004) Engaging families in health services research on childhood visual impairment: barriers to, and degree and nature of bias in, participation. British Journal of Ophthalmology, 06 2004, vol./is. 88/6 (782-7).

Ramaraj, R. and Chellappa, P. (2008) Cardiovascular risk in South Asians. Postgrad Med J. Oct;84(996):518-23.

Ranger, T., Samad, Y. and Stuart, O. (1996) Culture, Identity and Politics-ethnic minorities in Britain, Avebury, Aldershot.

Rapoport, R. and Fogarty, M. (ed.) (1982) Families in Britain, Routledge and Kegan Paul, London.

Raza, M. S. (1993) Islam in Britain, Past, Present and Future, (2nd edition), Volcano, Leicester.

Raza, Q., Doak, C.M., Khan, A., Nicolaou, M. and Seidell, J.C. (2013) Obesity and cardiovascular disease risk factors among the indigenous and immigrant Pakistani population: a systematic review. Obes Facts. 2013;6(6):523-35.

Richters, J. and Khoei, E.M. (2008) Concepts of sexuality and health among Iranian women in Australia. Australian Family Physician, 03 2008, vol./is. 37/3(190-2).

Riggs, E., Davis, E., Gibbs, L., Block, K., Szwarc, J., Casey, S., Duell-Piening, P. and Waters E. (2012) Accessing maternal and child health services in Melbourne, Australia: reflections from refugee families and service providers. BMC Health Services Research, 2012, vol./is. 12/(117).

Robinson, F. (1993) Separatism among Indian Muslims the politics of the United Provinces Muslims 1860-1923, Delhi, Oxford University Press, London.

Rose, E.J.B. with Deakin, N., Abrams, M., Jackson, V., Peston, M., Vanags, A.H., Cohen, B., Gaitskell, J. and Ward, P. (1969) Colour and Citizenship, Oxford University Press for Institute of Race Relations, London.

Sajwani, R.A., Shoukat, S., Raza, R., Shiekh, M.M., Rashid, Q., Siddique, M.S., Panju, S., Raza, H., Chaudhry, S. and Kadir, M. (2009) Knowledge and practice of healthy lifestyle and dietary habits in medical and non-medical students of Karachi, Pakistan.J Pak Med Assoc. 2009 Sep;59(9):650-5.

Shaw, A. (1994) 'The Pakistani Community in Oxford', in R. Ballard (ed.), Desh Pardesh: The South Asian Presence in Britain. Hurst, London.

Simmons, D. and Williams, R. (1997) Dietary practices among Europeans and different South Asian groups in Coventry. Br J Nutr. 1997 Jul;78(1):5-14

Simon, C.M., Zyzanski, S.J., Durand, E., Jimenez, X. and Kodish, E.D. (2006) Interpreter accuracy and informed consent among Spanish-speaking families with cancer. Journal of Health Communication, 07-08 2006, vol./is. 11/5(509-22), 1081-0730;1081-0730 (2006 Jul-Aug)

Skjonsberg, E. (1982) A Special Caste? Tamil women of Sri Lanka, (2nd edition), Zed, London.

Taylor, J. (1976), The half-way generation, a study of Asian youths in Newcastle-Upon-Tyne, NFER, Windsor.

Thomson, M.D. and Hoffman-Goetz, L. (2011) Challenges of recruiting ESL immigrants in to cancer education studies: reflections from practice notes. Journal of Cancer Education, 03 vol./is. 26/1 (170-4)

Twinn, S. (1997) An exploratory study examining the influence of translation on the validity and reliability of qualitative data in nursing research. Journal of Advanced Nursing, 08 1997, vol./is. 26/2(418-23).

Tziomalos, K., Weerasinghe, C.N., Mikhailidis, D.P. and Seifalian, A.M. (2008) Vascular risk factors in South Asians. Int J Cardiol Aug 1;128(1):5-16.

Ulvi, O.S., Chaudhary, R.Y., Ali, T., Alvi, R.A., Khan, M.F., Khan, M., Malik, F.A., Mushtaq, M., Sarwar, A., Shahid, T., Tahir, N., Tahir, Z., Shafiq, S., Yar, A. and Alam, A.Y. (2009) Investigating the awareness level about diabetes mellitus and associated factors in Tarlai (rural Islamabad). J Pak Med Assoc. Nov;59(11):798-801.

Visram, R. C. (1986) Ayahs, Lascars and Princes, Pluto Press, London.

Vydelingum, V. (2000) South Asian patients' lived experience of acute care in an English hospital: a phenomenological study. Journal of Advanced Nursing, 01 July 2000, vol./is. 32/1(100-107).

Warraich, H.J., Javed, F., Faraz-Ul-Haq, M., Khawaja, F.B. and Saleem, S. (2009) Prevalence of obesity in school-going children of Karachi. PLoS One. 2009;4(3).

Wasay, M., Khatri, I.A. and Kaul, S. (2014) Stroke in South Asian countries. Nat Rev Neurol. 2014 Mar;10(3):135-43.

Watt, I.S., and Howel, D. and Lo, L. (1993) The health care experience and health behaviour of the Chinese: a survey based in Hull. Journal of Public Health Medicine, 06 1993, vol./is. 15/2(129-36).

Wellock, V.K. (2010) Domestic abuse: Black and minority-ethnic women's perspectives. Midwifery, 04 2010, vol./is. 26/2(181-8), 0266-6138;1532-3099.

Werbner, P. (1990) The Migration Process: Capital, Gifts and Offerings among British Pakistanis, Berg, Oxford.

Yeowell, G. (2010) What are the perceived needs of Pakistani women in the North west of England in relation to physiotherapy, and to what extent do they feel their needs are being met? Physiotherapy, 01 September 2010, vol./is. 96/3(257-263).

Yildiz, C. and Bartlett, A. (2011) Language, foreign nationality and ethnicity in an English Prison: Implications for the quality of health and social research. Journal of medical Ethics, 10 vol/is. 37/10 (637-40)

Zakiullah, M., Muhammad, N., Khan, S.A., Gul, F., Khuda, F., Humayun, M. and Khan, H. (2012) Assessment of potential toxicity of a smokeless tobacco product (naswar) available on the Pakistani market. Tob Control. 2012 Jul;21(4):396-401.

Zaninotto, P., Mindell, J. and Hirani, V. (2007) Prevalence of cardiovascular risk factors among ethnic groups: results from the Health Surveys for England. Atherosclerosis. 2007 Nov;195(1):48-57.